A
Beautiful
Medicine

Praise for *A Beautiful Medicine*

"In our overstressed lives, we need heavy doses of renewal. When the neuro-endocrine consequences overwhelm our physical, mental, emotional and spiritual wellbeing, we need something more than antibiotics—we need something transformational and transcendent. Kerouac with *On the Road* and Pirsig with *Zen and the Art of Motorcycle Maintenance* each inspired a generation and guided a movement. David Mercier's marvelous book will do the same. After reading this engaging integration of stories, philosophy, and medicine, you will never think of healing in the same way again!"

> Distinguished University Professor Richard Boyatzis, Ph.D.,
> Departments of Psychology, Cognitive Science and
> Organizational Behavior at Case Western Reserve University;
> co-author with Dan Goleman and Annie McKee of the international
> bestseller *Primal Leadership* and co-author with Annie
> McKee of *Resonant Leadership*

"In his remarkable book, *A Beautiful Medicine*, David Mercier has described revolutionary new ways of understanding disease, health, and healing. It is beautifully written, well researched, and a treasure trove of transformative ideas. His therapeutic strategy transcends the conventional allopathic interventions; it treats the symptom not as a pathological phenomenon that needs to be controlled, but as a message that can lead us to the deeper roots of the problem. He weaves a rich tapestry of medicine, psychotherapy, acupuncture, diet, exercise, spirituality, and art. Illustrating the efficacy of this multidimensional mosaic are touching, compelling personal stories from his practice. By emphasizing the importance of meaning in human life and moving beyond distorting illusions about our own nature and the nature of reality, David Mercier combines the roles of therapist and spiritual teacher."

> Stanislav Grof, M.D., author of *Beyond the Brain, Psychology of the*
> *Future, The Cosmic Game,* and *When the Impossible Happens*

"*A Beautiful Medicine* is the best prescription for a longer, healthier, more satisfying life that I've ever encountered. It makes total sense. It gives you hope. It's uplifting. If you care about your health and well-being–your quality of life–you should read this important book."

> Roger Vaughan, author of *Herbert Von Karajan; Ted Turner—the Man*
> *Behind the Mouth; The Grand Gesture;* and others

A
Beautiful
Medicine

A Radical Look at the Essence of Health and Healing

DAVID MERCIER

Still Pond Press

Disclaimer

The information in this book is not intended or implied to be a substitute for professional medical advice, diagnosis, or treatment. All content contained in this book, including text, graphics, images, and information, is presented for general information purposes only. The author and publisher specifically disclaim all responsibility for any liability, loss, or risk, personal or otherwise, which occurs as a direct or indirect consequence of the use and application of any of the material in this book.

Grateful acknowledgement is made to the following publishers and authors for permission to reprint:

From The Universe is a Green Dragon by Brian Swimme. Copyright © 2001 by Brian Swimme. Reprinted by permission of Inner Traditions. www.InnerDirections.org.

From THE HOUSE OF BELONGING by David Whyte. Many Rivers Press, 2010. Copyright © 1997 by David Whyte. Reprinted with permission of David Whyte.

From The Essential Rumi. Translations by Coleman Barks with John Moyne. Copyright © 1995 by Coleman Barks. HarperCollins, New York. Reprinted with permission of Coleman Barks.

"Harlem (2)" from THE COLLECTED POEMS OF LANGSTON HUGHES by Langston Hughes, edited by Arnold Rampersad with David Roessel, Associate Editor, copyright © 1994 by the Estate of Langston Hughes. Used by permission of Alfred A. Knopf, a division of Random House, Inc.

From Talks with Ramana Maharshi. Copyright © Sri Ramanasramam. Reprinted by arrangement with Inner Directions, Carlsbad, CA. www.InnerDirections.org.

From Man's Search for Meaning by Viktor E. Frankl. Copyright © 1959, 1962, 1984, 1992 by Viktor E. Frankl. Reprinted by permission of Beacon Press, Boston.

Reprinted with the permission of Scribner, a Division of Simon & Schuster, Inc., from I AND THOU by Martin Buber, translated by Walter Kaufman. Copyright © 1958 by Charles Scribner's Sons. Copyright renewed © 1986 by Raphael Buber and Simon & Schuster, Inc. Translation copyright © 1970 by Charles Scribner's Sons. All rights reserved.

"The Seventh Elegy," "As Once the Winged Energy of Delight," copyright © 1982 by Stephen Mitchell, from THE SELECTED POETRY OF RAINER MARIA RILKE by Rainer Maria Rilke, translated by Stephen Mitchell, translation copyright © 1980, 1981, 1982 by Stephen Mitchell. Used by permission of Random House, Inc.

Excerpt from "Little Gidding" from FOUR QUARTETS copyright 1942 by T.S. Eliot and renewed 1970 by Esme Valier Eliot, reprinted by permission of Houghton Mifflin Harcourt Publishing Company. World rights, excluding U.S., and electronic rights granted by Faber and Faber, Ltd.

Cover photo: Water Lily, © Tomohiko Sugimoto 2011. All rights reserved.
Cover design: Metze Publication Design and Eclectic Graphics
Interior design: Metze Publication Design
Triptych photo—third portrait: Richard Dorbin. Triptych photo editing: André Mercier

Library of Congress Control Number: 2012934215
ISBN-10: 0985242507
ISBN-13: 978-0-9852425-0-3

With all my love
to Phoebe and André

Table of Contents

Acknowledgments

The word that comes to mind as I think of all the people who have contributed directly or indirectly to the existence of this book is the word *ubuntu* from the African Bantu dialect. Roughly translated, it means, "I am what I am because of who we all are." I'm deeply grateful both to those who have contributed throughout the years to my personal growth and to those who have directly helped this book evolve into its present form. The book is what it is because of who we all are.

First, my gratitude to the monks at Kanduboda in Sri Lanka for their tireless devotion to my meditation practice during my stay there a long time ago. Ven. Sumatipala Nayaka Thera, Ven. K. Seevali Thera, and Ven. G. Pemasiri Thera were beacons of wisdom and selflessness, and I am deeply grateful for their guidance and support during my years with them.

Stanislav Grof, M.D., has been a guide and teacher whose brilliance is matched only by his compassion. Stan, thank you from the bottom of my heart for your great kindness, your insights and methods, and your lifetime of research—all of which have benefited so many people throughout the world. Your work has reached more deeply into the roots of my life than anything else I've ever experienced, its impact profound and permanent. I will always be grateful for your invaluable contribution to the trajectory of my life.

Lynne August, M.D., is a radically insightful physician whose work in nutrition has had a most salutary effect on my health throughout the years. Thank you, Lynne, for your tireless exploration of the clinical gems you find beyond the mainstream, and for the caring you always bring to your work, to me, and to your patients.

Michael O. Smith, M.D., D.Ac., founded the Lincoln Hospital Recovery Center in the South Bronx, New York, which was responsible for treating up to two hundred drug addicts a day for about thirty-five years. Mike, thank you for your endless generosity of time and energy in supporting my projects throughout the years. I'm grateful for your spirit of service to the world. It has helped sustain my professional growth and contributed to a number of successful initiatives.

Dianne Connelly, Ph.D., L.Ac., and Bob Duggan, L.Ac., founded the Tai Sophia Institute, where I first learned about the basic principles of health and healing that serve as cornerstones for this book. Dianne and Bob, thank you for your courage, humor, and pioneering spirit in bringing forth the wisdom of the healing traditions. Your contributions to my life through your work and our friendship are only one small part of your broad legacy. I continue to value our long-lasting friendship.

Stephen Blood, D.O., is a wizard in osteopathic manipulative medicine. Dr. Stephen, thank you for your healing hands and for being a true master of your craft. Your rare gifts have been of great help to me over the years.

A warm thank-you to my professors at the Weatherhead School of Management at Case Western Reserve University: Richard Boyatzis, Ph.D., Harlow Cohen, Ph.D., David Cooperrider, Ph.D., Ron Fry, Ph.D., Eric Neilsen, Ph.D., and Melvin Smith, Ph.D. In my eyes, your frequent ranking as the best Organizational Behavior department in the world is well deserved. Your pronounced influence on my life has in part led to this book; the blend of your intellectual strengths with your ability to care deeply about the human condition will continue to be a great inspiration to me.

On the winding road to the book's final form, many people offered their support by critiquing the first draft. For that, a big thank-you to Anne Adams, L.Ac., Mary Brandenburg, L.Ac., Bonnie Kasten, and Roger Orsini, M.D. In particular, Dick McCauley and Jane McCauley graciously devoted a good deal of time offering their astute observations and suggestions. I thank you all not only for your suggestions, but for being enthusiasts for the book. All your comments lent new angles and perspectives that helped shape it into its final form. I extend my deepest appreciation to all of you for the precious time you gave to the early version of the manuscript. It could not have continued to develop without your help.

Bruce McGraw and I were on the phone once a week for a year and a half, coaching each other on writing our respective books. Thank you, Bruce, for your insight and perspectives on both the contents of the book and on the process of writing. You often saw what I couldn't when my nose was to the grindstone. Your support throughout the writing of this book was invaluable, and I'm very grateful.

Ronald Sieber and Cate Collins, thank you for the clarity and optimism you provided during the publishing leg of the journey. I value our collaboration and have greatly enjoyed the fruit of our conversations.

Thank you, Sue Loweree, Del Joiner, and Patty Joiner for your ongoing support, encouragement, and enthusiasm while I was immersed in writing. It was delightful.

To Kippy Requardt, an enormous thank-you for editing the book, for your command of the language, your eagle eyes, and your excellent job of editing the book into its final shape. A special thanks also to Roger Vaughan for his advice and encouragement along the way. I'm deeply grateful to you both for your skills.

To Tomohiko Sugimoto, thank you for your generosity in providing the exquisite photograph on the cover.

To my patients, thank you for sharing your life stories with me. Over the years, I have learned about the deep essence of our shared humanness as I listen to your descriptions of the pain of illnesses and the joys of healing. Your trust in me and your honesty have contributed more to my life than you will ever know.

To my long-deceased parents, Jean-Marie Mercier and Joko Homma Mercier, the word *gratitude* can't express what I feel for your devotion to me during the time you spent on this planet. I miss you and I always will.

And to my children, Phoebe Harding and André Mercier—what jewels you are in my life. Thank you for being you. I wish you nothing but the best to be found in heaven and earth.

Introduction

In 1975, when I was twenty-three, I flew to Sri Lanka and became a Buddhist monk. After shedding my long wild hair, electric guitar, blue 1958 VW Beetle, and everything else I owned, I settled in for two and a half years at a monastery called Kanduboda near the hamlet of Delgoda—a hot, rickety bus ride from Colombo and worlds from America. Hoping to recapture the serenity and elation I felt after a couple of month-long meditation retreats in California, I sold everything I owned and staked my all on this one, big gamble.

The elation I'd felt was more than just good vibrations—it was waking up bolt upright, becoming fully alive and wide-awake conscious. After the retreats, I could feel in my bones the meaningfulness of knowing I was bonded, in some ineffable way, to the sky, to the earth, to all the others who walked the face of the planet. I felt calm, free, clear—bathed fresh in clear waters—and more spirited than I'd ever been in my life. It was as intoxicating as it was unfamiliar. I sensed, for the first time, that some new voice at the boundaries of earth and sky was speaking to me in sure tones, calling me forward and mapping the next steps in my life. I felt a beautiful stillness that lay like a soft blanket on my often-troubled self. Best of all, everything started to add up. The puzzle of being human seemed easy to piece together for the first time in my life, and the big picture began to make sense. After the retreats, I knew that I wanted nothing more than to pursue the mystery of these vast, invisible worlds I'd glimpsed. It seemed that destiny had come knocking.

But I'd soon be disappointed to feel the effects of the retreats dissolve after a few months, to find my self-doubt and moodiness returning in full force like a repeat thunderstorm. Then, all I wanted was to meditate more and restart the engines of my deliverance.

After discussing options with my American meditation teacher, we decided I would go to Sri Lanka, where he had been a monk and where I could meditate for as long as I wished.

Kanduboda was set into a plantation of tall, leaning coconut palms, fronting a macadam road with the occasional ox-cart or rusty car ambling by. It was a humble place befitting the monastic traditions, and with its collection of one-story outbuildings, simpler than temples in the cities like Colombo and Kandy. Foreigners often came because it focused more on the results of meditation practice than on the study of the old texts and because they were welcome to stay a week or two in retreat. When I arrived, I had no money or possessions left, and no way home. I trusted that when it was time to return— *if* I were to return at all—I'd find a way. If I liked my new surroundings well enough, who knew—I might want to stay there all my life.

After meeting the monks and getting oriented on my first day, the muscles in my face were sore from smiling. Since the old Buddhist books are gloomy in spots, I hadn't expected radiant faces. The monks beamed like sapphires. Though only a few of them could speak English, we bonded instantly through our shared task of working on what was most meaningful to us. Surrounded by orange robes, shaved heads, and a smile flashing in every corner of Kanduboda, I felt right at home.

I was assigned a small room in the meditation building, where I would live for the next two and a half years. My five-by-eight foot cell had a smooth concrete floor and plaster walls; at night, I slept on a thin coconut husk mattress on the concrete sleeping platform a few inches high. Over the next year, I occasionally exchanged the three-inch mattress for a thin tatami mat, which meant essentially that I was sleeping on concrete. I did this to see if it would help reduce my attachment to comfort, a move that would have won the approving nods of a few ancient *arahats*, or fully enlightened ones. It didn't last.

A few months after I arrived, I was ordained a *samanera*, or novice monk. I'd come with the intention to meditate for five or six years, hoping that if

I worked hard enough at it, I'd become immune to the pains of the human heart. After all, this was the promise held out by the ancient books mapping the way to complete liberation, bliss, and freedom from suffering. It appealed to me as a member of the disillusioned counterculture looking for a new social order after the debacles of Watergate and Vietnam, and more personally, as a young man who had been plagued by self-doubt, melancholy, and a brooding uncertainty about how and where I belonged in the world. The idea of nirvana, either literal or figurative, fit well with my full enrollment in the romanticism of the sixties and the ethos of Woodstock, fed by news of the Beatles' trip to Rishikesh and the exhortations by Ram Dass to Be Here Now.

In the meantime, my friends back home wondered why I'd trade the comforts of the flesh for such an austere life—no music, no food after midday, no sex, no contact with women, no money, no entertainment, and, not insignificant to a hippie, no hair. My answer was that exchanging all that for the smooth contours of a peaceful mind, not to mention the occasional all-natural rapture, was a bargain. What I wanted most was to make these changes permanent, to have the steady, resolute heart I'd always found elusive.

But shortly after beginning my first meditation retreat in February, something went awfully wrong. I developed a crushing pressure between my eyes and on my forehead, and from that moment on, I was unable to concentrate. The sensation wasn't a pain, but an enormous, brute pressure—a pushing, as though someone were shoving a bowling ball into my face. Eventually, this led to some sort of short-circuit in my brain: I couldn't think, I couldn't focus, and within a few weeks, I was suffocating in a morass of depression. If trouble meditating were compared to difficulty in keeping my attention on a flower vase in a room, what I experienced was the darkness that follows turning off the lights. I couldn't see a thing. I couldn't even make out what I was supposed to focus on—much less stay concentrated on it.

Over the next two years, the pressure became heavier, thicker, more tangled. Before long, it devoured me. My brain and my thoughts turned as dense as the dark jungle surrounding Kanduboda, my moods as murky as the tropical nights filled with spider, snake, and scorpion. Within a year, I became suicidal. I had staked my all on this adventure—I had nothing else on which my identity could rest—and I'd lost, alone here on the other side of the planet, far from the support of my family and friends. I thought that the best way to end my life would be to wander into the surrounding coconut plantation and get bitten by a cobra. If it looked accidental, my parents back in northern Virginia might have found my death a little less painful.

When I arrived in Sri Lanka, I was about six feet tall and weighed just under a hundred and sixty pounds. After a year and a half, I was down to a hundred and twenty pounds from malabsorption in my small intestine and from two types of intestinal worms. My ribs stuck out like the rows of a corrugated roof. Medical tests at a hospital in Colombo showed that my small intestine's villi— the thin filaments that absorb nutrients—were badly damaged. This meant the nutrients in the searing hot fish and vegetable curries, red rice, coconut, and tropical fruit weren't getting into my bloodstream. As a result, I became anemic and malnourished. Between the malabsorption and the worms, I was at the doorsteps of starvation even while eating prodigious amounts of food. Twice a day in the dining hall, local devotees put as much food as I wanted in my black metal alms bowl, but to no effect. I couldn't gain weight.

In the meantime, the pressure and the depression worsened. Despite my best efforts and the expert instruction of my teachers, I was becoming weaker, more brittle, more depressed. All day, every day, I felt this twisting, crushing pressure driving into my face, head, and brain—I felt as though its tendrils were pressing into my cranium itself. As a result, I became so confused that on occasion I had trouble following a conversation between two people. At other times, the pressure around my head and neck was so strong I had trouble speaking.

When I first arrived at Kanduboda, I did a nine-month retreat during which I'd meditate all day, every day. The retreat involved waking up at four in the morning, then alternating between sitting cross-legged in silence for an hour and walking for a half-hour. This went on until ten or eleven at night, a routine punctuated only by breaks for personal hygiene, a short meeting with my meditation teacher, and the two meals of breakfast and lunch. Rules for the monks included fasting between noon and the following morning.

After the nine-month retreat, I was worse. Later, I did retreats of two and three months' duration, but the pressure remained. In the past, meditation had left me feeling calm and clear, but now, I was a walking calamity. I remember being crushed with envy when other monks and laypeople would show serene, shining faces after just a week or two of meditation.

Finally, after struggling with this from February 1975 until June 1977, I was on the verge of collapse. I knew that if I kept it up, I'd snap like a wooden board pressed too hard, and I began to consider returning home. My teacher Pemasiri Thera and I had agreed to put a stop to my preparations for full ordination, which would have meant following over three hundred rules of the order. I was too sick to endure a more rigorous routine.

The chief monk, my teachers, and all the other monks encouraged me to stay, as monkhood was the most substantial of lives, and in Buddhist countries, the noblest. I loved my monk friends, the sensitivities of Kanduboda, the warmth of the Sinhalese people, the smart, funny, beaming Pemasiri Thera, and the kindness in the eyes behind the coke-bottle lenses of the chief monk, Venerable Sumatiphala Nayaka Thera. But I felt that I had no choice but to turn in my robes. I had to get back to the U.S. to regain my health and protect my sanity.

After my father sent me money for the return trip, I got on my way in June 1977. I first stopped in Madras (now Chennai) and then Calcutta (now Kolkata) for brief stays. After seeing the cruelties of poverty as I walked the streets, I thought about staying in India, maybe to help Mother Teresa. But I was so sick and depleted that if I had, I'd have gotten sicker. Or worse.

I then went to Burma, long before it became Myanmar, where I asked for the advice of the Venerable Mahasi Sayadaw in Rangoon. I spent a week resting in Bangkok, spent time in Hong Kong, Taipei, Seoul, and then a couple of months in Tokyo with a cousin and her family before returning to the U.S. in October 1977.

After returning, my recovery was slow. While conventional medicine got rid of the worms while I was still in Sri Lanka, my doctors back home were unable to find any reasons for the pressure. So I began a long exploration of other types of therapy: acupuncture, chiropractic, osteopathic manipulation, nutrition, herbs, supplements, massage, and more. I was in psychotherapy for a long time. I went to personal growth workshops. Over the next several years, as I regained weight and began to feel normal, the pressure improved marginally. But though the symptom itself stayed strong, I rebounded and became healthier overall during those years. I kept using all these therapies well after becoming an acupuncturist in 1983. In the decades since, by being the beneficiary of these therapies myself, I learned firsthand a good deal about them and about the merits of natural healing.

The struggles during my years at Kanduboda have led roundabout to the lessons contained in this book. All I have learned about healing and natural therapies has come out of the ashes of the devastation I experienced in the green, teardrop-shaped island in the Indian Ocean. A twist or two of fate, and I've been privileged with a lifetime of witnessing, from the front row, the wellspring of healing at work. I never intended to get into the health professions—being a rock star looked more glamorous in my teen dreams—but my illness and depression in Sri Lanka led me straight into one with a legacy of about three thousand years. Throughout the book, I'll describe more about my own healing journey to illustrate the principles of health and medicine laid out within these pages.

After nearly three decades and over thirty thousand patient visits, I feel fortunate to have peered deep into the heart of the healing process itself. Time and time again, I've observed in my patients what leads us to vitality and vibrancy, and what puts us on the highway to misery—and it's this that I want to share in the book. With these insights in hand, I trust that you'll be better equipped for the decisions about health and wellbeing that you and all of us will face at some point in our lives.

The world of integrative medicine has been variously called complementary, alternative, natural, and holistic. I've chosen to describe a way of looking at health and medicine that I'll call *a beautiful medicine*. While it overlaps these natural healing approaches, it's more. It's more than a different set of techniques.

What is a beautiful medicine?

It will take the whole book to describe the idea, but a preview may help. A beautiful medicine is about going beyond, while including, the mechanical, biological view of the human body. It embraces the soft underbelly of our humanness along with the outer shell of hard scientific data. It holds out a vision for medicine that respects the soul and spirit at the core of human experience. When art and science—the subjective and objective—are combined, we have the makings of a richer medicine, a more complete picture. For example, by understanding a person's sorrows, loves, fears, and dreams, we have more coordinates for pinpointing the diagnosis. This helps us treat not just organs and other body parts, but the living, pulsing soul of a human being. It's a humanistic medicine, but as we'll see, it's also much more.

In the end, we want more than just knowledge and information. We also want a result with feeling, with the textures of joy and passion. No one wins a championship game and feels blasé; no one makes a breakthrough scientific discovery without a thrill, and the end of all our search, we hope, is not a bland, insipid place but one of gratification—with a feeling, a tone, a mood. Similarly, at the end of our lives, most of us would like to sigh with the satisfaction that we've lived a life worthwhile, not to go out with a shrug. But whatever form it takes, it's a feeling—not just a flicker in our brains, but a flush of warmth in the heart and soul. I'll attempt to show throughout the book that folding our search for fulfillment into the biological puzzles of the body can lead to a richer understanding of health and healing. Health is as much about the condition of our souls as it is about our physiology.

Behind the statistics on disease, behind scientific theory, we find, always, the soul of the human narrative. We find there the scent, texture, and flavor of our humanness: the stench of anguish, the perfume of euphoria, the wounds of trauma, the sweat of sexual ecstasy, the leaps of jubilation. We are thirsty to live freely, to live unbound, or, at the least, to get by with a little less trouble and a little more peace. But today, soul and science are divorced. In our view of the body, we've excluded the Shakespearian conundrums and the long trail of sorry tales that fertilize the roots of illness.

Today, we get our reminders about the primacy of the heart and soul from the screen, stage, and printed page. It's art, not science, that reminds us of those quiet places within where the heart opens wide like an almond blossom in the spring or cracks from the iciness of grief and disappointment. That's because the soul often goes incognito behind the flesh. In its enchantment with science and technology (as exciting as they are), with flurries of math equations, Hadron colliders, smartphone miracles, and stealth fighters, science easily forgets about the soul—those places within where we *feel* most deeply. When a shoulder or leg or gut becomes an ambassador conveying the message that anguish is percolating in the soul, we concentrate on what's most palpable—the proverbial squeaky wheel. We act like Nasruddin, who looked for his house keys under the lamp post—that's where the light was, so he looked there even though he'd lost the keys further up the street. The lament of the aching body plays at louder volumes than the whispered voices of the soul. We are drawn to what we can see, touch, measure. It's easier.

But in the end, science and soul can be eminently good partners. A medicine that is whole and beautiful will include both of them. Throughout the book, we'll see why that's important. In many instances, the real incentive for some patients in seeking professional help may be the need to be touched, seen, heard, known—to remember that *I am*. The body's grievances just so happened to get them to the clinic of a solicitous human being who might serve as a *de facto* lover, father, mother. Or an archetypal one. So a good working hypothesis for the health professions would be that behind every symptom is an unabridged human drama that's been percolating for years and then appears at this one sore spot on the body. The symptom looks like an unexpected intruder, but it has been lurking behind the scenes for years, fed by stress, unhealthy food, too little sleep, paltry amounts of exercise, and a life skewered by disaffection. As we'll see, sometimes a knee pain is just a knee pain. Not all symptoms and illnesses are connected to troubles in the soul. But often, and very often, they are.

This broader, more inclusive vision of health includes ideas that have been handed down to us for centuries or even millennia. Many of those insights from ancient traditions are still relevant today, an enduring legacy of the power in wisdom—not knowledge, but wisdom: the capacity to see deeply and clearly. Long before the invention of the microscope and the telescope, the ancients were analysts of nature's patterns. They observed how nature worked in both the physical world and in the mind and body. They felt in their bones an intimacy with the winds and the earth, the sun and the moon, the trees and the oceans. Everything they could possibly experience, including medicine and healing, planting and harvesting, hunting and cooking, was another face of the one revered cosmos.

Over the centuries, these ancients engineered medicines from plants and animals. They found, for instance, that some herbs helped with headaches and others with menstrual cramps. Nearly 5,000 years ago, the Ayurvedic medical tradition of India found therapeutic value in turmeric, a spice used in curry. Today, medical research has shown it to be a strong antioxidant, possibly useful as a protection against cancer. Ancient Chinese medicine found many uses for ginseng, which today is considered an adaptogen—a substance that supports our resilience in times of stress. The ancient Egyptians and Persians, as well as Hippocrates in Greece, discovered the makings of aspirin in willow bark over 2,500 years ago. Over time, all these ancient healers created an impressive pharmacopeia.

Throughout the book, I will not write much about research or about specific healing methods, but about the deep patterns of healing. There are plenty of other resources on methods and research. And although I practice acupuncture, I won't describe it other than to touch upon it briefly in stories about my patients.

Instead, I want to convey something beyond tip, technique, recipe, and formula: it's the charisma of this magnificent vitality of existence running through our veins. It sings, hums, and growls in the human body, sculpting and being sculpted by the vignettes of our personal dramas. I don't think I can define healing, but the stories you'll read, and the ideas behind them, may help you better feel its presence.

As an acupuncturist, I've had the privilege of listening year after year to people tell me the stories of their lives—formulas for failure, recipes for vitality, costs of fear, joys of courage, pain of unspoken secrets, rebirth out of the ashes. It has given me a precious glimpse into the core of healing as well as the heartbeat of the soul. While the stories vary, there seems to be only one pulse throughout: the heaving and thrusting of the energy of life itself. If we look *through* the symptoms instead of *at* them, this breathing, pulsing current of aliveness reveals itself, leaving us more awake and more alive, touched by the fingertips of an unseen grace. It will help us get plugged into nature's nerve endings, to step one bit closer to whatever it was that created nature.

Once you understand the basic ideas of healing, you can apply them in a variety of situations. For that reason, this is not a how-to book, though I have waxed practical at times. Instead, it's a look at the essence—the deep, core principles—of health, healing, and medicine. These principles are by definition abstract, but they are to my mind essential. I have tried my best to illustrate them as concretely as possible.

I hope the book leaves you better informed for the job of making the best choices you can for health and vitality throughout your life. If you know how to drive, you can get to your destination in nearly any car. Similarly, I hope that the principles contained in the book will help you navigate the confusing ocean of healthcare choices. The idea was expressed by the sixteenth-century Swiss doctor Paracelsus when he wrote:

Medicine is not only a science; it is also an art. It does not consist
of compounding pills and plasters; it deals with the very processes of life,
which must be understood before they may be guided.

So I prefer to convey ideas about the very processes of life rather than to provide prescriptions like which acupuncture points relieve headaches or which herbs are good for insomnia. It's not about the techniques of integrative medicine, usually called complementary and alternative (CAM), nor about which medicines or methods are best. It's about demolishing the calcified beliefs about health and healing that are rapidly becoming decrepit with age.

Some of the ideas you'll read about are so unlike our usual notions of health that they may surprise you. I expect this because virtually every patient of mine is surprised, even startled, by many of them. Our usual notions of health are ones we've swallowed whole, not because of any defective thinking, but through cultural habit. We grew into them from childhood, absorbing them through the currents of culture like a towel soaking up water. Just as we don't have to consciously think about which side of the road to drive on, we don't question the conformist views of health and healing, views which then become unquestioned reality.

All this is directly related to the crisis in our healthcare system which is buckling under the weight of flawed designs and concepts. But most relevant here, the system is floundering under the misplaced assumptions about what health is in the first place. While it's a given that we must get to the roots of a disease, that means different things in different camps of medicine. Much of our healthcare budget is spent on everything but digging up those roots. In addition, the healthcare system is just beginning to see the gasping obviousness and peerless logic of preventing illness and fostering optimum wellness. Prevention makes far better sense than costly tests and treatments for a disease that didn't need to happen.

One foundation for this book is the vision that health is more than the absence of disease, and medicine more than remedial work. While this has long been advocated by the World Health Organization as well as many physicians and most practitioners of integrative medicine, it simply hasn't taken hold yet in our culture. This new vision for health is about being fully alive and vibrant, being juiced with meaning and purpose, and being at home with our spiritual nature—a condition suggested by Saul Bellow interpreting William James: "People really lived when they lived at the top of their energies." So it's not only about the integration of mind, soul, and body, not only about hardiness, vitality, and the thump of a good heartbeat. It's also about being immersed in the oceanic wisdom surrounding us, about finding our rightful place in the world, coming to roost in our authentic existential home. It has to do, as cosmologist Brian Swimme wrote, with "becoming the mind and heart of the planet," where we step beyond the limitations of a life circumscribed by an undue allegiance to a "me" and exploring what lies beyond the self as we know it. This broader picture includes what's called the transpersonal, the academic translation of what we'd usually call spiritual.

I hope the book helps rearrange, perhaps make topsy-turvy, your perspectives on health and healing, and leaves you at least one bit healthier, if not changed at the core. I wrote it with the intention of consolidating what I tell my patients in fragments from session to session, trusting it would be more useful when packaged. As for its intended audience, I'll go by the words of e.e. cummings, who once said he didn't write poetry for "mostpeople." He wrote poems for only you and me.

Chapter One

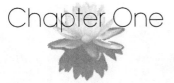

The Spirit of Medicine:
The New, the Old, and the Beautiful

Health is not just the absence of disease, but the flourishing of human possibility. It's a spark between hearts, tears of forgiveness, fires of love, good bones, strong muscles, belly laughs, a blush in the nerve endings of the soul. It's about thriving, blossoming—all of it driven forward by the deep human yearning that choreographer Martha Graham called *the blessed unrest*, by what Goethe called *the holy longing*. Health is more than a freedom *from* disease: it's license *for* being wholly alive. By itself, it goes transparent like a shoe that fits perfectly. We don't want it for its own sake, but for what it allows us to do. We'd never think of going into the living room to just sit there and be healthy for an hour. We want health *in order to, for the purpose of*...it sets us free to play soccer with the kids, make love, work hard, paddle a canoe, inhale the scent of the small angel cuddled in our arms.

Our current model of health and medicine works remarkably well in many ways, but it's biased: it has been seduced by the brilliance of hard, sparkling data in the scientific pursuit. In contrast, the ethereal aspects of human experience, like beauty and soul, often go dim before our glowing achievements in technology and science. It's humbling to look up at towers of steel and glass or to board a giant jet and then wonder about the place of soul and spirit in all this. The miracles of science and technology, in spite of their abuses and limitations, have clearly improved lives in remarkable ways.

They're fascinating, and most of us are grateful. But it helps to know when they catalyze human potential and when they obscure it.

With medicine, our culture has grown accustomed to engineering the body. We shape, control, and manipulate it as we might a car engine. But if we listen to poets, philosophers, and the ancient healers, the body is far more than a contraption of flesh, bones, and other pieces: it's a prism for immeasurables like beauty, love, and wisdom. In their view, the body is not a thing but the insinuation of a deeper truth—it's a 3D representation of mysteries we've taken too literally, a screen projection of the creative forces hiding behind the extroversions of life. Plato wrote of this in his allegory of the caves: we've spent so much time in the cave of our perceptions, he said, that we mistake the shadows on the wall for reality. We've forgotten that what's real are the flesh-and-blood people standing outside the cave, and that of all the mysteries in heaven and earth, the human body is only one measurable, tangible, and huggable part. One of the most compelling descriptions of this idea comes not from a great philosopher, but from Judy Garland. In her 1939 book of poetry, she wrote:

> *For 'twas not into my ear you whispered, but into my heart.*
> *'Twas not my lips you kissed, but my soul.*

And dancer Isadora Duncan said:

> *The dancer's body is simply the luminous manifestation of the soul.*

While we now have reams of studies about the mind-body connection to support these sorts of ideas, it's still hard for our research community to shake off the allure of tangibles and the habit of peering only through the looking-glass of science. In the predominant view, it all revolves around scientific validation, which will pass final judgment on whether or not something is real.

Today, our culture has seen the early emergence of a new vision for medicine and health that leaps beyond that sort of thinking. This new vision respects the ineffable poetry that animates the human body. It considers the body not a mechanical assemblage, but a fountainhead of the world's audacity. This poetry, reaching in from places invisible, inhales and exhales the body.

Yes, energy comes from mitochondria, those power plants in the cell that give us fuel for our bodies' engines. But then, how did mitochondria get here in the first place? Too much has been written in theology, philosophy, and our spiritual traditions for us to summarily dismiss any notions about the indiscernible as the whimsy of indulgent minds. But to our culture, trading in the currency of tangibles feels more secure, as it's far easier to touch a tree than a forest. Seeing health and medicine in an integrative light requires opening the doors of perception and searching for the invisible projector showing the movie. It requires increasing our respect for the abstract, for the invisible, for the ethereal vapors of love and wisdom, to better see how they are infused into flesh. Science goes in the opposite direction by purging bias and belief out of its experiments—rightly so, but at a price if we stop there. Although poetry and scientific research have been strange bedfellows so far, that's beginning to change. It's an opportune time, given the crisis in healthcare, to recapture the holism and lyricism in medicine found among the ancient Persians, Indians, Tibetans, Greeks, Native Americans, and Chinese, and to let them permeate the citadels of science. The doctors of those times were poets, artists, athletes, priests, and philosophers—and to them, the body was not just a compilation of fingers, bones, and organs, but an integral part of the universe's script. The gods were in on it too. From the ancient Persian text of the *Vendidad* in the *Avesta*, dating back probably to 800 B.C., we find:

Of all the healers O Spitama Zarathustra,
namely those who heal with the knife, with herbs,
and with sacred incantations,
the last one is the most potent as he heals from the very source of diseases.

–Ardibesht Yasht, Vendidad

In one of the cornerstones of ancient Chinese medicine, the *Huang Ti Nei Ching*, from about 400 B.C., we find:

When the minds of the people are closed and wisdom is locked out,
they remain tied to disease....it becomes apparent that those who
have attained spirit and energy are flourishing and prosperous,
while those perish who lose their spirit and energy.

To think of the human body as just a biological contraption is to think that a Matisse or O'Keefe is a bunch of paint molecules—true, but incomplete, and therefore misleading. The love, beauty, and inspiration that decorate the interior of our lives ask for a bigger explanation than the firing of brain cells. While specialization has merit—you wouldn't want your plumber to also be your marriage counselor, and vice versa—we need to remember the relevance of the part to the whole. In recent decades, medicine has started to show more interest in blending the different faces of the human experience into a workable whole.

When patients are given time in the treatment room, they often rush headlong into reading aloud from the storybook of their lives. As in a play or the work of investigative journalism, their stories include a full cast of characters caught in a messy plot that ends with the symptom as headline. It's a drama uniquely theirs, revealing a story that often sounds like the work of a scriptwriter run amok. If we were to equate real with relevant, these narratives are often more real than that herniated disc or that heartburn. This doesn't negate the science or ignore the symptom. It includes both while looking through and beyond them, searching for all that's relevant.

As consumers of healthcare, we usually want, in the end, more than just to have our bodies repaired. We want a partner as we learn to flourish. We want our bodies repaired *for*...for the freedom to live as we wish. With this in mind, integrative medicine sees the patient's montage of stories as context for health and illness, and helps her piece her life together, sometimes reassemble it, into a poem that flows in rhyme. That rhyme can include the yearning to belong, to be financially secure, to chuckle more, to be wholly loved, and in short, to have a life existentially full and satisfying. As we look at what we as patients need, we want both body and soul vibrant. We ask for help fixing our knees, and we also want our stories to be heard. Science and soul can be excellent dance partners.

> No artist is pleased. There is no satisfaction whatever at any time. There is only a queer, divine dissatisfaction, a blessed unrest that keeps us marching and makes us more alive than the others.
>
> –Martha Graham

The notion that health goes transparent is one starting point for an integrative model of health. If health's value lies in the freedom to live as we wish, health professionals face the starkness of an existential question: what are they ultimately doing in medicine? Well, for one thing, they can fix broken parts. Or they can do the necessary repair work and *simultaneously* help the patient flourish, to become fluent in a vocabulary that nurtures heart and soul. This is essential. Self-expression is healthy: it clears the heart of clutter. Confidence is healthy: it eases the jumpiness of fear and the zing of adrenaline. Serenity is healthy: blood flows better calm. Fluency is healthy: smooth is better than rough and bumpy. Clarity is healthy: decisiveness heals better than ambivalence. If the health professions were less distracted by the shadows on the cave wall, they could redefine their mandate as midwifery for the birth of human possibilities.

Physics tells us that about 13.9 billion years ago, nothing at all existed. Then, in a massive, fiery explosion, we suddenly had a universe with hydrogen and helium. Spurred by other big explosions over the eons, new elements later came into existence. Over time, to make a long story very short, they became you and me. The carbon, hydrogen, oxygen, and other elements in our bodies today are simply new shapes of the exact same elements that make up hundreds of billions of galaxies, each with hundreds of billions of stars, many of which are billions of light years away. As an indisputable fact of physics, we are, literally, stardust.

The ancients could feel in their veins this intimacy with the universe. Though they knew nothing of stardust or the Big Bang, they could sense oneness just as we can smell the ocean when we draw near. So they revered it and built temples of belief and tradition in its honor. Using both observation and intuition, the Native Americans, Egyptians, Persians, Indians, Chinese, Greeks, Tibetans, and many other ancients pre-empted the current research on the mind's effect on the body through the discovery that sacred incantations had power. They respected the grandeur of the spiritual empire concealed behind water and fire, wind and earth. They bowed to the magic tucked inside the blue hills and green valleys.

Today, medicine would do well to reclaim its place in this grandeur. A doctor or other health professional examines a sick patient in an office in a town in a state in a country on a planet in a solar system in a galaxy in a universe. Medicine as a whole can likewise remind itself of its contexts—it always occurs in context—and insinuate itself back into the big picture by asking questions of meaning, purpose, reverence, metaphysics. At the least, it would be more invigorating and satisfying for all involved. At the most, it could transform medicine. In the existential question of what health professionals do, being repairmen is no longer enough. Since broken hearts are often hiding behind the broken parts, medicine's job should include restoring the heart's romance with its origins, the soul of aliveness itself. Medicine's strategy could include, among other things, helping a lost, isolated self find its way home to rediscover its primal intimacy with the world. Mystics have been telling us for centuries that we're not separate from anything else and that we're just different faces of the one same universe. The heart aches when we don't see that. As the poet David Whyte wrote:

There is no house like the house of belonging.

When we feel alienated, resentful, envious, or lonely, we're stuck in what the Hindus call *maya*: the illusion that we've disaffiliated from the divine play, the Whole, which, in their eyes, is impossible. Piercing this illusion brings us closer to fulfilling the unwritten promise of our lives, and in the end, this should be a purpose of medicine.

It seems a long distance between these ideas and, say, the whir, glint, and clatter of machines in a shock trauma unit. But it isn't. If we look past these machines and the people running them, we'll find the primordial impulse to preserve life and that deep, silent mystery lying behind the veils.

Chapter Two

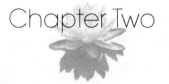

Symptom as Message

A symptom is a message. In the final sense, it is not an aberration, but the perfect articulation of a summons to change. It intends only the best for us. An allusion to its rightfulness lies in Walt Whitman's line, "And I will thread a thread through my poems that time and events are compact. And that all the things of the universe are perfect miracles, each as profound as any." His idea that everything is a perfect miracle helps in redefining a symptom as the sound of nature's honest and eloquent voice, as a directive guiding us with its wisdom. Although this idea is radically different from our usual opinions of these uninvited and aggravating guests, it can transform, at the core, our approach to health and to the art of living. We have much ground to cover, but I'll start with a story about Olivia.

Olivia (all patients' names are fictitious) was a tall, dark-haired woman with a quick smile and a sharp sense of humor. She sought my help for menopausal hot flashes, insomnia, a brooding anxiety, and a few pains here and there. The aftereffects of several unhappy relationships, plus the stress of a questionable one of the moment, also weighed on her. But of all her symptoms, what stood out for me was the pervasive, jittery discomfort of her anxiety.

During her third visit, I suggested that she think of her anxiety not as a problem, but as a message. She could then redefine it as a visitor with a good purpose: it was only trying to help her. I talked about how her sympathetic nervous system, the fight-or-flight response, was stuck in high gear. While it usually kicks in when there's danger, whether real or perceived, it can get stuck on red alert. As unpleasant as it feels, its original purpose was charitable: it had given her the surge of energy needed to run or to fight danger. Our bodies evolved through the millennia to rely on a temporary shot of energy to fight off a saber-toothed tiger or to run from the spears of marauding cavemen. In response to a threat, this source of energy would be available even without the usual energy derived from food.

As we redefined her anxiety as a survival tool, Olivia quickly understood the logic. Nothing in her life today warranted these feelings, so we could assume they came from her past. While she no longer needed this sort of self-protection and while she didn't know its origins, it would help if she understood that its intentions were good. At the least, it would reduce her aggravation about the sensations, which itself is another symptom.

After we finished talking, I had her lie on the treatment table as usual, and I began inserting a few needles. Within a minute, and though she barely felt the needles, she burst into tears and started sobbing loudly. It was a flood unleashed.

Acupuncture can evoke neurochemical changes that occasionally lead to a release of emotions, and, in Olivia's case, the needles combined with our conversation had triggered this flood of grief. As I put my hand on her arm and let her speak through her tears, a torrent of information poured out. She said she knew when she first started having this horrible feeling: she had felt it as a child every night after getting into her bed whenever she stayed at her grandfather's house. She would panic because she knew something awful would happen later when her grandfather came into the darkness of the room. While she had no memories of what took place, she knew without a doubt she was terrified to sleep in his house. She said she now understood her lifelong difficulty in falling asleep: danger might creep in through the door, so she needed to stay awake. She sobbed and told her story until her tears gradually subsided.

When we spoke on the phone the next day, Olivia said she felt great. After her treatment, she had gone to a meeting that would normally have left her tense, but her breathing had been markedly deeper, slower, and more relaxed. We had never discussed her breathing before. She said that after waking up that morning, she felt wonderful. The morning sun was exceptionally bright and the sky over the snowy fields a deeper blue than she could remember. Her body felt soft and calm, her sinuses had cleared, and she felt renewed. As a result, Olivia made long-needed changes in a work partnership, her finances, and her personal relationships. She was freer to jump in and better engage with the challenges of her life. When she opened up to her feelings and when she trusted the wisdom behind them, the anxiety began to release its hold on her.

The idea is simple: a symptom is here to help. It's telling us to change something somewhere. It's not a problem—it points to the problem, to the underlying distress or disease in the body, the mind, or both. Because that's such a departure from how we usually think of symptoms, the idea can be puzzling at first. But as we'll see, the idea can be pivotal in putting you on a healthier, happier course for the rest of your life. It can be life-altering.

This is a straightforward, conventional idea with implications poorly understood in our culture. One dictionary defines a symptom as "a characteristic sign or indication of the existence of something else." So the very definition of a symptom is that it's just a sign or an indication. The idea isn't new. It's widely accepted in the world of integrative therapies, from acupuncture to naturopathy and everything in between, where the symptom is respected as an inflection of nature. The idea dates back thousands of years through the ancient healing traditions—respected not only in the traditions of the East, but in the work of Hippocrates and his colleagues in ancient Greece. Though this is the definition of a symptom in conventional medicine as well, the prevalent methods of our healthcare system don't reflect this view.

Symptom as information

A symptom is information. By definition, it's a sign, and not the problem itself. As the Zen saying goes, when someone points to the moon, don't look at the finger. While the idea is obvious, and even a tautology (a statement like "my sister is a female"), it's new to every patient I see. Though it may be a bit startling at first, it's easy to understand eventually. But our instincts have told us otherwise: the symptom's discomfort seems proof that it's the enemy. We view it as kindly as we would a thief in the house.

The symptom is a red alert, a warning bell, a siren, a bullhorn, a flashing light on the car dashboard, the wailing of a smoke alarm, a baby's cry in the night. It's a whisper from the mystery in tree roots, an insinuation from the wisdom in the waters and the earth, intimations from the luminosity of the body. It's a notice, a dispatch, a wink, an omen, a clue, a communiqué, an urgent look from a colleague across the conference room. As strange as it may sound, it improves quicker once it earns your respect instead of your disdain. As provocateur, it wants you to change for your own good—whether by taking more potassium and calcium, eating less sugar, forgiving your mother, drinking less, eating more greens, or any of a huge number of actions. As the bearer of news, its strategy is benevolent. All it wants is the best for you. And if you don't shoot the messenger, you get more details.

If, as Whitman wrote, all things in the universe are perfect miracles, then symptoms too are perfect miracles. If your hand hurts when too close to a fire, the pain leads to the excellent solution of withdrawing your hand. Your nerve endings worked exactly as designed, precisely as planned, and you responded as they wished. What was "wrong" was being too close to the fire and risking damage, not the pain itself.

To better understand the intentions of a symptom, we need to stay alert to what's behind the scenes. The symptom is an exhibitionist, grabbing the spotlight while the director and playwright stay out of sight behind the stage. The symptom always points elsewhere: to nutritional deficiencies, viruses or bacteria, inflammation, the roots of anxiety, an unresolved past, or any number of conditions. For instance, the chest pains of heart disease are not the problem, but signposts leading us to the blocked arteries that reduce blood supply to the heart. If the pains were the problem, doctors would give narcotics to a patient with a heart attack just to ease the discomfort. Instead, the patient receives medications that relax the arteries, improve the flow of blood, and reduce stress on the heart.

My mother, who was Japanese, always shuddered at the rumble of thunder and the crackle of lightning. One night during the later years of her life, we were talking in her kitchen over a cup of green tea when a lightning storm struck. When the rumbling and crackling started, I saw the usual anxiety enter her soft brown eyes, as well as a self-conscious look that said, Isn't this silly that I'm afraid. But with every shockwave of sound, her small body trembled. Then that night for the first time, she told me why she reacted this way. The sounds reminded her of exploding bombs. As a seventeen-year-old girl, she would run in the night with her mother and sisters to air raid shelters where they huddled in terror as fire bombs from B-29s fell on Tokyo and the city burned down around them. After fifty years, without forgetting, her body was still ready with adrenaline to help her run like a frightened deer.

To heal from the core, we need to understand the symptoms, not subjugate them. Just turning down their volume through denial, overwork, drugs, alcohol, sweets, or machismo hurts us in the long run. All our therapies— whether herbs, medications, nutritional supplements, acupuncture, or massage—can be used either in coordination with, or in opposition to, the strategy of a symptom. To help illustrate the nature of symptoms, here's an analogy—one I will refer to often throughout the book.

The Story of the Broken Window

Imagine a man with a stressful job in a rough, competitive workplace. He's anxious about his performance, irritated with a few colleagues, and worried about being laid off. Imagine further that he feels tense, unwell, and fatigued, mostly from ignoring basic needs such as adequate sleep, rest, exercise, and healthy food. In addition, he drinks too much alcohol and coffee. Then, peering into his past, we see that he often fought with his father during his childhood. This affected his self-esteem, which in turn led him to put too much pressure on himself about his performance at work. To this day, he and his father have not reconciled.

On top of it all, his marriage is strained. His wife considers him self-absorbed; he considers her demanding. She feels the strain of trying to be supermother, superwife, and superexecutive. Like her husband, she ignores her needs for rest and self-care out of her obsession to perform slavishly at work. In addition, she's resentful that he's not doing his fair share of household chores. She also eats poorly, doesn't exercise, feels drained at the end of the day. She's worried about her mother, whose health is failing and who demands her love and attention but irritates her with every phone call.

Their teenage son has been unruly; he's doing poorly at school and has recently been rude to his parents who are, of course, remarkably out of date and jail-guard strict. The three of them have had shouting matches in recent months.

Next, imagine this husband and wife coming home exhausted one day to find that the son has thrown a party instead of going to school. The house is trashed. They yell and swear at each other, after which the son stomps into the den and, using a baseball bat, smashes a window. Then, imagine this argument repeating itself, for various other reasons, week after week for a while. Each time, there's another broken window.

One thing is obvious: this family does not have a window problem.

But that's how we think about our symptoms. We think the broken window, like fatigue, stress, headaches, and pain, are problems. But when you have fatigue, you don't have a fatigue problem—in the same way that this family doesn't have a window problem. Since the fatigue, or aches, or any symptoms at all are fingers pointing to the moon, we shouldn't be fooled by their vociferous tones. If you have constant headaches, you don't have a headache problem. The headache is *part of the solution* because it's an insistence, a demand, that something somewhere be changed. It demands action that will help you heal at the core.

As observers, the neighbors see only broken windows. Similarly, the symptom in the spotlight is the only visible sign of trouble. But behind those broken windows lies a complicated family history with subplots reaching out like the bare winter branches of an old maple tree.

Now, if we think the broken window is the problem, we could respond in a number of ways. For one, we could buy stronger glass to better resist the blows. We might double the thickness of the glass, use bulletproof glass, or install hard polycarbonate. We could search for the best repairmen, those with the most experience and the best track record. We might also want to find those charging the lowest fees for the best work, the best cost-benefit ratio. Then we'd want quick access, and we'd look for someone who will be available when we need him.

The analogy illustrates how we can think of our individual health and how we use medical care. But, to put it on a broader scale, we can also apply it to our healthcare system and see how it's designed largely to treat broken windows. If we think the country has a broken window problem, we could, for example, work to keep down the costs by buying our glass in bulk, hoping for a discount on volume. As for insurance, we could shop for the policy with the best coverage with the lowest deductibles for the best price. If we pooled our risk by becoming a big conglomerate with the neighbors, we could negotiate with the insurance companies for lower rates. Then, for prevention, we could bolt steel bars across the window or even replace the window with brick. Additionally, we could remove all baseball bats from the house.

These are the kinds of efforts we make when trying to improve our healthcare system. Clearly, they don't get to the core of the problem. We certainly need to repair the window to keep out the cold and heat. And windows are often broken by the blows of poverty. But in our current healthcare model, we have focused on repairing broken windows without looking into the source of the symptom. Given that perhaps 75 percent (some even say 90 percent) of chronic illnesses are preventable through lifestyle changes, this analogy is relevant to a hefty percentage of our healthcare costs.

It's certainly logical to say that the bat was the cause of the broken window. But then, we could blame the boy's hands, since they wielded the bat. But then again, the boy was upset by the argument, so we might say his temper was the cause. But then the parents might not have yelled if they'd been calmer. That would have been more likely if...on and on and on. We could trace events endlessly into the past to find many *streams of influence* converging onto that spot where the bat made contact with the glass. Consequently, the idea of a "cause" of illness, in many circumstances, is too simplistic. While there are illnesses with a single identifiable cause, like HIV, malaria, and so on, most illnesses are the tail end of many streams of influence.

As we work toward understanding health and disease better, we need to find not just the nearest cause of illness, but its roots—not only the last domino to fall, but the first. Repairing only the glass is too simple a response to an event that is one point of attachment in a complicated spider web. If we would instead look at the big picture, we'd have a better chance of getting well. Of course, the ambiguity of it all is a big challenge—with so many influences, we might not know where to begin or where to end. It can be a healing whodunit requiring the skills of a detective. To illustrate the complexity, the following diagram points to the variety of influences that can contribute to the onset of symptoms, directly or indirectly.

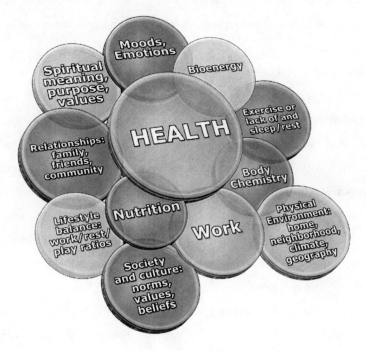

For Olivia, her anxiety was just the broken window. We shouldn't be fooled by the symptom's peskiness and its greed for being center stage. After all, that is the role it was assigned. Using herbs, acupuncture, or medications just to have her relax would muffle the message when what she needed most was to understand and heal the source of her anxiety.

The tragic death of Michael Jackson also illustrates the value of understanding symptoms. Reports indicate that Michael died when his doctor injected him with an anesthetic—a powerful drug for use during surgery, not at all intended as a treatment for the insomnia Michael suffered. But in light of our discussion here, we can see that Michael's insomnia was not a problem: it was a message pointing elsewhere. Who knows—it might have pointed to adrenal stress from rehearsals for the big London concert, emotional turmoil, the use of stimulants, or other factors unknown to us. But whatever they were, they led to the insomnia. Another approach would have been to find and eliminate the causes of his insomnia instead of sedating it, instead of patching up the broken window.

One day, Karen, who had started with me a couple of months earlier for chronic pain, came for her eighth appointment. (I will sometimes leave out specifics about symptoms, as their unique nature may identify the patient.) The unrelenting pain had begun a year and a half earlier after surgery, and since then, she'd had dozens of medical consultations with no luck. Most recently, she was at last finding some relief through a combination of acupuncture and medications. When she came for the appointment, she was free of the pain, and had not been bothered by it in recent days. On this day, after two months of becoming more familiar with me and the treatments, she was ready to reveal more about herself.

During the previous weeks, Karen and I had discussed nutrition, exercise, and general health matters as well as her family stresses. She suspected these stresses were feeding her pain. But on this day, secrets came pouring forth like a mountain stream. You could almost sense the impulses of life pressing forward to unburden themselves, to find release, purification, and closure as she spoke. She talked of being terrified as a young girl during her father's alcoholic rampages. In his drunken rage, he'd pummel her mother and her brothers in front of her. Though he'd spared Karen, witnessing the violence petrified her. Her father's drunkenness was poisonous to the emotional arteries of the family and scattered its toxic waste among all of them for years.

Since those days, Karen had come to believe that her father drank to drown the heartbreak of having seen many of his fellow soldiers, good friends, killed during World War II. She said he never talked about it. To add to the stresses, an older brother sexually molested her for three years starting when she was seven. In addition, she had been assaulted regularly, both physically and verbally, by her boyfriend for seven years when she was a teenager. As if that weren't enough, she wept as she spoke about her fear that God was angry at her, that she was a religious failure. As she told her story, her pain suddenly kicked up again for the first time in days. It was the broken window. We will come back to Karen's story later.

The layered symptom

Smith Island, Maryland, is a small community with a big reputation. With a little over three hundred people, the island struggles to survive as the harvest of crabs, oysters, and fish from the Chesapeake Bay dwindles and as thousands of acres erode back into the water. But it's also known throughout the state for its signature confection, a cake made of up to fifteen layers of alternating cake and frosting.

Like a Smith Island cake, symptoms are usually layered. They have many facets. Just as the cake layers aren't contradictions of each other, neither are they mutually exclusive, so the different dimensions of a symptom fit together in a coherent whole. Karen's pain was clearly the result of a physical procedure gone wrong, but the need for emotional closure took advantage of the spot's temerity. The layers of the cake can include structural, biochemical, energetic (the level at which acupuncture and homeopathy work), psychological, social, and spiritual dimensions. A key point here is that several or even all of them can contribute to a symptom simultaneously.

In contrast, we're accustomed to looking for the single cause of a symptom. It's the single-bullet theory: find the one cause, which will lead to the one remedy and then to the cure. In many illnesses, this is clearly the case: infectious diseases are caused by viruses or bacteria, and once the single invader is conquered by medication, the patient recovers. But even then, outbreaks of a disease like malaria must be seen in light of the social, economic, and political conditions of the country. The strength of the patient's immune system before infection, and the condition of her psychological wellbeing, must also be considered. If a country's budget is heavily weighted toward buying weapons, then the public health funding for the prevention and treatment of malaria will suffer.

The bottom layer of the cake represents the most primitive job of the symptom: it's there to help us survive. Over millions of years, our minds and bodies learned that great pain could signal death or danger. Duly noting exceptions such as the pain of childbirth, we saw the correlation: the worse the pain, the more it threatened life. So the impulse of survival communicated through urgent voices, telling us to change our behavior for our own good. In tandem with that, sensory pleasures usually led us to act in ways promoting strength, resilience, and fitness. Meat, berries, and roots were enticing when fresh, but repulsive when rotten. The pleasures of sex eventually led to larger families and clans, which then helped us survive and stay healthy. The sense of security, belonging, and strength—an asset in the struggle for survival—sat better in the human body.

But the other levels of the Smith Island cake represent the social, psychological, spiritual dimensions. They don't contradict each other; instead, they all contribute to the complexity of a symptom.

Restoring my own health

The messages from my own symptoms began to take shape after I returned from Sri Lanka to the Washington, D.C. area in 1977. They guided me as I began looking for ways to extract myself out of a black hole, the likes of which I'd never known.

When I first returned from Sri Lanka, the pressure on my head and face was still colossal and easily aggravated. I was also exhausted. At times, I'd feel drained after walking up one flight of stairs. When I went to have my teeth examined by the residents at the Georgetown University School of Dentistry, the only place I could afford, they found twenty-seven large cavities and four teeth that needed crowns. Since I hadn't eaten desserts during my time at Kanduboda, I suspect malnutrition was the culprit that laid waste to my teeth. During the period I had the work done, I spent an entire day in the dental chair several times.

I also had no trouble complying with the recommendations of my doctors in Sri Lanka to eat as much as I could. Being incessantly hungry and compelled to grossly overeat must have come from my having been drained to the point of starvation. I would stuff my lonely belly, sometimes eating for an hour straight, until I felt like a bloated carcass. Fortunately, I didn't gain weight because of my quick metabolism.

Since my doctor in northern Virginia didn't have a diagnosis for the pressure and didn't suggest any further evaluation, I started exploring complementary and alternative therapies, which, over time, all helped to restore my vitality, strength, and emotional wellbeing. But none of them, nothing, made a difference in the pressure itself. The symptom—my curse, as I saw it then—was to shrink by only the smallest of measures over many years.

Slowly, I became culturally acclimated back home, a now-strange world where everyone spoke English, no one bowed to the ground before me, no one stared at the rare white monk the way they had in Sri Lanka. Life here was a fidget, with far fewer signs of spiritual sensibilities than I'd seen during my travels in India, Sri Lanka, Thailand, and what was then Burma. Back home now, I was strangely out of place—the soul of a monk at the circus. While I'd quickly adapted to life as a celibate, penniless barefoot monastic in Sri Lanka, I would need years to readjust back home. Then again, the location of my cultural home was debatable—I was born in Japan and had lived there until I was fourteen.

My father had been deployed to Japan after the war as a soldier in the Army, eventually becoming a civilian accountant for the Department of Defense. Shortly after arriving, he met my mother, who was working as a secretary in his office building. When I was a child, our family lived on a housing annex not far from Tokyo called Grant Heights. Unlike bases such as the Air Force's Tachikawa with its airplanes and the Navy's Yokosuka with its battleships, Grant Heights was a residential enclave for military families. We lived in a small duplex with an Air Force colonel and his family in the other unit. The duplex backed up to the boundary of the annex, which I would often cross on my blue bike to the abandoned wooden shrine behind us and explore on my own other unknown territory for hours and miles. It was safe for a ten-year-old boy to just wander off into the countryside in Japan.

Between moving to northern Virginia in 1966, attending Annandale High School for a couple of years and spending four years at James Madison University (then Madison College), and leaving for the East, I'd been in the U.S. for a total of nine years. This meant that at the time of my return in 1977, I'd still spent fewer years in this country than I had out of it. When we first moved to Virginia during my sophomore year in high school, I was at sea. Here was a biracial kid from the genteel culture of post-war Japan and a buttoned-down, all-boys Catholic school now trying to fit into a high school with girls, and with kids who smoked, drank, and swore. It was all foreign and frightening to me. So with only a nine-year history in the land of the free, I wasn't sure when I returned after my monk years if I was readjusting or just learning to adapt for the first time. During my first week back, I walked into a supermarket. After seeing the thousands of colors and glaring lights,

I was so overwhelmed I rushed back out. Compared to the tranquil nights at a Buddhist temple with oil lamps and chanting monks, it was all Vegas to me. Rock music, the former staple of my cultural diet, at first sounded alien, almost sinister. I also learned the bad news that while I'd been away, disco had been born.

Before long, I learned that the pressure on my face and head would constrict or relax depending on the circumstances. When I was active, as in running or dancing, it would loosen. When I was still, it would squeeze and tighten. Whenever I sat in the meditation posture, the pressure would become monstrous, leaving me confused and gloomy for days afterward until it lifted on its own like fog at midday. After seeing this pattern consistently over the months, I got the hint: I was supposed to keep moving. It was a symptom, and its message was for me to move, stay active, extend my reach into society, and above all, not to sit in meditation—which I received in the same way Ella Fitzgerald or the Beatles might have received an injunction not to sing. Reluctantly, and with no small amount of shame at my spiritual failures, I put aside the contemplative arts and became active again: dancing, running, playing guitar, and moving about. My symptom was pushing me toward the life of the everyman, toward normalcy, toward the social mainstream with all its flaws and merits.

The pressure also contained psychological elements. On the one hand, while it would turn into a vise grip with physical triggers like doing yoga, drinking coffee, or sleeping in a car with my neck bent, it would also squeeze harder when I was tense or nervous. Like a Smith Island cake, the pressure was textured with both emotional and physical layers. Unfortunately, whether it was aggravated by a physical or emotional trigger, I'd sink to the bottom of a foul moodiness for several days before it slowly faded on its own. Being active and outwardly focused would clearly help it slacken. It was telling me to keep moving. And when I listened to the instructions, I would feel better.

After staying at my parents' house for a few months, I moved into a group house on Dahlia Street in Northwest D.C. with several other meditators. We thought that by living together we'd encourage one another's meditation practices and spiritual interests. Instead, we threw dance parties. But the dancing gave me insight—it reinforced the idea that I needed to literally and figuratively shake things up. The parties were wild, though not drunken, and we danced, exhilarated, until breathless and spent. During it all, I'd feel the pressure loosening up, however temporarily, and feel more like myself. Eventually, it became incontrovertible, regardless of my aspirations for a contemplative life: I had to relinquish the meditative quest and get busy, get active, and accept the possibility that a conventional life had merits. In Buddhist monastic terms, it was a householder's life—clearly second fiddle according to the ancient texts, but acceptable. The monks back at Kanduboda never disparaged it, but you could sense the implications about its failings by the phrasing of their words. I was ashamed to the core about this. Because of my lifelong insecurities, I had clung to the meditation as a panacea, a redemptive possibility that I'd hoped would catapult me into a more self-assured life. The one tool that had helped me feel strong and confident was now as distant as the northern tundra.

I remember how my first meditation retreats in Capitola near Santa Cruz, California, would leave my soul calm, my ears and eyes clear. The world looked unexpectedly beautiful; to suddenly find sunbeams of joy emanating from a shy and often melancholy young man was an unexpected bonus. It had all come from just closing my eyes, all day, every day, for a month, and meditating. So I concluded, mistakenly, that all I needed for my final emancipation from the melancholy and uncertainty was to go inward, stay silent, and be still. After all, the best methodology I'd had until then—sex, drugs, and rock and roll—hadn't produced such divine results. Monks in Himalayan caves, Thai forest hermitages, or Sinhalese jungle hideaways couldn't all have been fooled for the last twenty-five hundred years. Since they all did it, maybe it really was a formula for unparalleled peace, a quiet heart, and the end of discontent.

Only later would I realize that emotional maturity and social fitness were the lower rungs on my ladder of spiritual growth that I had skipped. The pressure on my head and face had clear intentions: it was telling me to start again at the bottom of the ladder, to engage face-first with the dribs and the minutiae, as well as the pleasures, of living in society. But then again, after a glimpse into the beauty and immensity of spiritual freedom, everything seemed minutiae. The challenge was to open my eyes wide enough to find grace, presence, and effulgence in the ordinary, even in the hollowness of social theater. I was to find, for myself, that society was a legitimate spiritual laboratory—not exactly a monastery, but for now, maybe even a better challenge for me than sitting on the meditation cushion. So the pressure was a symptom, which was a message. It was instructing me to move about, to get about, to laugh, play, joke, sing, and to take myself less seriously.

During the first ten years after returning from Sri Lanka, the pressure decreased only slowly. Fortunately, this was outpaced by my emotional growth and progress with my physical health. I graduated from acupuncture school, established a private practice, got married, and then got divorced after fourteen years, though I now have two lovely children out of that union who are the jewels of my life. Some years after the divorce, my ex-wife and I were able to laugh in agreement that each of us will live longer because we're not married to each other. Fortunately, we're good friends now, and I continue to adore her sisters and their families. During the years of inching my way back to normalcy, I was mowing the lawn on the riding lawnmower one hot, sticky day when I looked at the mower and then at the station wagon in the driveway. It hit me: I'm neither hippie nor monk anymore.

So in exploring the idea that the symptom is a message, we move on to consider the other layers of the Smith Island cake. While the symptom is rooted in the basic impulse for survival, it can simultaneously mean much more. We've looked at how the mind and body are like threads woven into each other, but beyond that, we also have the spiritual facets to consider.

A spiritual layer of the cake

A student once asked the revered Indian sage Ramana Maharshi how to manage the dissatisfaction of a life with no time left for spiritual pursuits. He was impatient to move on with his spiritual life, he said, but work and other obligations got in the way. Ramana Maharshi answered:

> The world is only spiritual. Since you are identifying yourself with the physical body, you speak of this world as being physical and the other world as spiritual. Whereas, that which is, is only spiritual.

The quote has never stopped echoing in my mind since I first read it many years ago. It's a beautiful reminder to always look beyond appearances, to see through the haze of the conventional. And with a similar view expressed in Walt Whitman's saying that each thing in the universe is as profound as any, we can then consider all symptoms in that light. If that which is, is spiritual, then ultimately, *every symptom is a spiritual phenomenon.*

Many ancient healers and mystics said we are an integral part of the cosmos, of the vibrant, pulsing energy of the world. Alan Watts echoed the idea when he wrote that we didn't come into the world, we came out of it. Among ancient cultures, the metaphors for a living spiritual force, a life force, were remarkably similar: *ruach* in Hebrew, *ki* in Japanese, *prana* in Sanksrit, *spiritus* in Latin, *qi* in Chinese, and *pneuma* in Greek—all of them referring to breath as the symbol of a life-giving cosmic force. It was the breath of the heavens arousing life on earth. In the West, French philosopher Henri Bergson wrote of the *élan vital*, or the vital impetus; German philosopher Arthur Schopenhauer wrote of the similar *will-to-live*; and Nietzsche wrote of the will to power. All these ideas suggest a universal life force that permeates the human body and all that exists.

So symptoms, just like anything else in the world, are the indelible expressions of this life force. As voices of life's energy, they're equal to love, beauty, ecstasy, and other such experiences in their legitimacy—certainly not in their desirability—but in their validity and in their being a stakeholder in your wellness. Symptoms are not aberrations, but smart, useful, and meaningful incentives directing us forward. They're communications from the professors of wisdom residing in body and mind, from the pulsing of a self-organizing current of aliveness that encourages us to flourish. This pulsing is at work whenever we get the urge to sing, pray, dance, rest, or sleep. But it's also there even in the simple act of breathing in and out, when our noses itch, when we're bored or enthusiastic, when we're sleepy, when we feel great after a workout, when we're happy to be in a beautiful dress or on a fast motorcycle. It speaks to us directly, every second of our lives, in every and any sensation we experience. Whether pleasurable or not, sensations, urges, and drives are not static and inert like rocks; rather, all are part of a vast orchestrated aliveness.

The message of a sensation can be clear, when, for example, a stiff back says we've been standing too long or too wrong. Or it can be complicated, when stress is encouraging us to forgive and let go even when our pains come from being victimized by an assailant. Or it can be simple but obscure, such as when fatigue tells us in code that we need more vitamins and minerals.

But the message can be even more nuanced and textured. Pioneering psychiatrist Stanislav Grof, M.D., Ph.D., has written about the way our personal struggles can result from a *coex*, or *system of condensed experiences*. A coex, like a Smith Island cake, is a pattern with many layers and without a single cause. Claustrophobia, as one example, might have several origins. The phobia may have roots in a stressful experience in the womb, caused by the mother's own stress. Then, in a difficult delivery, the baby may have gotten stuck, leading to feelings of entrapment. (Grof and other psychiatrists like Freud's disciple Otto Rank have long asserted that *in utero* experiences affect human development, and only recently has this idea begun to gain acceptance in academic circles.) Then the trauma of being locked in a dark closet during childhood might add still another layer to the claustrophobia cake. As a teen, a terrifying experience of being stuck in an elevator complicates the matter even further. Together, all these experiences can contribute to the fear of enclosed spaces. In this hypothetical case, the patient has no single cause for claustrophobia, but a complex bundle of influences.

In my own life, the work of Stan Grof and his wife Cristina have been of seminal importance as I sought to peel back the claws of the pressure on my head, face, and soul. Their expressive techniques took me to the dark, deep layers hidden well below sight lines, to where I found the serpents coiled at the base of my spine. Over a period of two years, through fourteen full weeks of explorations in the unconscious, through the bellow and roar of all that my spirit needed to express, and also through the visions of beauty and possibility that sometimes left me weeping in joy, the pressure began to release its clutches on my head for the first time. I saw the coex at work: my symptom was deeply spiritual and archetypal, plainly psychological, but it was also physiological—a cup of coffee would set it off. This wasn't strange, as I'd thought initially, but proof of its complexity. Over time, the healing that came to me from Stan's work has been precious beyond words.

It's transpersonal

The spiritual and physical dimensions of the human experience are an integrated whole. With that as a backdrop, we can redefine the essence of a symptom as not just a voice of biological impulses but as an expression of life's evolutionary thrust.

To explain this, let's start with a simple look at pain and pleasure. Both have existed in organic life forms for millions of years before we were born and were included in the original plans. This capacity to feel is an inheritance, a dictum that existed long before any of us as individuals came along. We had nothing to do with the fact that we feel pain or pleasure, and it's far more than our individual subjective experience of sensations. A child in Tibet, a warrior in the Amazon, a grandmother in Ghana, or a banker on Wall Street are all beneficiaries of this capacity for pain and pleasure, however uniquely their subjective experience is molded by culture and history. Ultimately, we can think of symptoms as transpersonal events, which means, stated a bit too simplistically here, that they're ours but simultaneously more than that: they're also part of a larger universal script. Symptoms are the progeny of a wisdom trailing fourteen billion years into the past and indefinitely into the future. They're the exclamation of life's intelligence, of the world's blueprint, of the electricity lighting up the entire universe.

The moment you feel pain or pleasure in your body, you're feeling the prodding of nature's brilliance. It's the very power that moves the sun and moon, that brings us calf and colt in the spring, that makes the leaves go brown in October and green in April. That breath of life swirling along the axis of creation and destruction across endless time and space is the same power that produces pain and pleasure at the nerve endings of your skin. The sensations aren't void of meaning, nor are they happenstance. They're voices of the ineffable orchestra of the Whole, singing even through the slightest ache or the slimmest pleasure. It's life itself speaking to life—a surging, swelling, heaving energy that's as alive in a steel mill or a skyscraper as it is in bucks and does drinking from a mountain brook. Sensations are intelligence—they're the handwriting of life as it comes to know itself through our particular eyes and ears, skin, nose, and tongue. In the *Art of Contemplation*, Alan Watts wrote, "The individual is an aperture through which the whole universe is aware of itself." He tells us that each of us is the center of everything around us, not as separate beings, but as particular expressions of the Whole. Each of us, he says, is how the universe becomes aware of itself. If we accept this, we are much bigger existentially than we usually seem to ourselves.

Symptoms are then part of this design—they're expressions of the Whole, even while they seem to belong to only you. So our symptoms are not, as we're inclined to think, pointless or haphazard nuisances. On the contrary, they're articulations of the great wisdom of life itself. And if we respect the symptoms as such, we can take our cues and respond accordingly instead of ignoring, resenting, or fighting them. Brian Swimme writes, "To become the mind and heart of the planet…is to…live in an awareness that the powers that created the Earth reflect on themselves through us." The genius of nature's architecture embraces pain and all symptoms.

Watts and Swimme and others have written that we are more than isolated, physical specks in the grand order of things. They tell us we are woven into the Whole, in a song that mystics of Christian, Hindu, Buddhist, Sufi, Jewish, and indigenous traditions have been singing for millennia. In this view, then, every cell in the body and every sensation we feel is part of a grand, universal design. Seeing symptoms in this way revolutionizes their meaning: they're opportunities for seeing our intimacy with the power that created the Earth reflecting on itself through us.

In the Native American traditions, this idea was prominent. From the Pawnee tribe, we have this:

> *In the beginning of all things, wisdom and knowledge*
> *were with the animals, for Tirawa, the One Above,*

did not speak directly to man. He sent certain animals to tell men
that he showed himself through the beasts, and that from them,
and from the stars and the sun and the moon
should man learn...all things tell of Tirawa.

–Eagle Chief (Letakos-Lesa)

In the 1990s during a visit to the Santa Clara Pueblo in New Mexico with my family, I met a young medicine man with clear steady eyes and a shiny black ponytail that fell to his waist. In his twenties, he was apparently one of the youngest of his tribe ever to have been designated a medicine man. As we talked, I was struck by how mature and poised he was for his age—he spoke with the authority and wisdom I'd have expected from an elder. You could see a long way into his eyes. As we compared the ancient Chinese and the Native American views on medicine and healing, we noted the similarities. Both views emphasized the inherent healing potential in the body. Both diagrammed human physiology with the symbols of nature like earth, water, and fire. Both thought of healing and medicine as reflections of the spiritual powers of the universe.

With this in mind, we can redefine our symptoms as elements of our spiritual unfolding. We think they're obstructions, when instead they can be a part of the spiritual journey itself. They're not in the way: they *are* the way.

There's an old joke about a pastor in front of his church who is approached by a fire truck as floodwaters rise. The firemen encourage him to come with them to safety, but he refuses, saying, "The Lord will save me." Later, after the waters have reached halfway to the roof, men in a rescue boat come by, also encouraging him to come with them. He refuses again, as he says from a second-story window, "The Lord will save me." The floodwaters then reach even higher, and as the pastor stands on the roof, he waves a rescue helicopter away, shouting, "The Lord will save me." But the waters continue to rise until he eventually drowns. Once in heaven, he confronts God angrily, saying, "I believed in you. I trusted you. How could you let me down?" God answers, "I sent a fire truck, a boat, and a helicopter. What more could you want?"

Listening to the messages

We usually resent the fire trucks, boats, and helicopters sent our way. We resist them. This is understandable. As Charlie Brown once said to Lucy, "Pain hurts." But resenting a symptom stuffs our ears with cotton just when listening to the message is crucial. Ironically, the tension that comes from feeling victimized by or antagonistic toward the message only amplifies suffering. Conversely, acceptance helps—not resignation, acquiescence, submission, or inaction, but a creative willingness to embrace the truth of their presence. Pain is different from suffering. Pain is a sensation in the body or mind, while suffering is pain amplified by the commotion of emotions. The melodrama of fear, worry, and anger only intensifies the symptom. It's possible to have pain and not suffer—not that it's common or easy—but it is possible.

We have become impatient with symptoms by two routes. One is the primal instinct to pursue pleasure and avoid pain—which won't change because we're born with it. The other is the cultural drift toward quick fixes and the dogged pursuit of easy gratification. On the air, on the web, and in print, we're deluged by ads encouraging quick pleasures and easy solutions. Whether they offer solutions for depression or hay fever, or formulas for the perfect life, the underlying message is that comfort and pleasure are a cultural holy grail. Not only are these messages found in advertisements, they're implicit in everyday conversation, in unexamined assumptions, in the cultural air we breathe. However subliminally, the messages leave their impressions on us like handprints in clay. Nowhere do we find encouragement to reflect on the meaning of symptoms, and everywhere we find tips, tricks, and tools for eradicating these pesky nuisances without delay. The symptom gets no respect.

Since no one naturally defaults to seeing a symptom as a message, the idea must be learned. It's a concept foreign in the lands of the instinctual, primal brain. Unfortunately, the normal instinct to eradicate symptoms without understanding their implications is not harmless. In the long run, it can make us sicker. If we ignore the very messages guiding us toward health, we might discover the roots of the illness too late. If instead we remember that the symptom's intentions are admirable, we can become its respectful, cooperative partners. For all their annoying or devastating effects on our lives, we can remind ourselves that they're collaborators. Understanding this can transform your life.

Depression in another light

To illustrate this point, a quick look at depression may help. In the language of everyday culture and in that of the clinic as well, depression is a disorder needing treatment. It's a problem, with a diagnostic code, and it needs repair.

But we can look at it in an entirely different way by considering it a symptom, a finger pointing to an unseen moon. Whether the depression is bothersome or devastating, it's always a message, not the problem. This is a crucial distinction to keep in mind. You might find it strange, as depression can devour us like the whale of Jonah and spit us back out. But the cloying, painful distress of depression is an incentive—it's precisely what pushes us to understand ourselves better, to heal deeply, to free ourselves from the shackles of a troubled emotional past and from neurochemical distress. The discomfort itself is precisely what presses on us to uproot the source of the depression. The message may be to purge painful memories, to respect ourselves, to love fully, to stop eating sugar, to forgive, to know that we are loved. If we cooperate, we'll have discovered a profound source of strength.

Our usual view is that depression is a disorder, an illness, and the result of a serotonin deficiency. Granted, some depressions are mediated by a serious chemical imbalance and may benefit from pharmacological help. But even they, the most serious of depressions, are messages. Most psychotherapists look for the deeper roots of the depression, but in the world of medicine, the focus is mostly pharmacological. For some people, a boost of serotonin through anti-depressants may help. But a chemical deficit in the brain is the cause of depression in the way the baseball bat was the cause of the broken window. It was the weapon that made contact with the window, but many other streams of influence trailed behind it. These include the neurochemical, historical, cultural, racial, familial, genetic, psychological, financial, and spiritual dimensions of the person's life. With every depression, we have a unique person being prodded by an impetus to grow, to exorcise the demons of the past, to learn to love more, to be assertive, to be bold, to nourish the body beautifully, to be able to say *I am*, to blossom, to flourish. Depression hurts, but calling it a problem is an exercise in interpretation, not a description of an inherent truth.

For people with mild to moderate depression or with a normal, appropriate sadness, anti-depressants are today often prescribed by rote, given without considering all the influences that could have led to the symptom. Sadness at the breakup of an intimate relationship or from the death of a spouse is normal and natural. What's there to fix? Those feelings are simply a normal expression of our humanness, a necessary exertion of the human experience. Only if a person did not feel sadness would something be wrong.

To take this even further, grief is a teacher. It can lower us into the deepest, most authentic places within and pull the gates of the soul wide open, where we can find a compassion and empathy more delicate than before—if we choose that route instead of cynicism. As arrogance and grief rarely coexist, being brought to our knees by the brute hands of grief or humiliation can help us become more sensitive to the pain of others. Our souls will become softer if we welcome grief as mentorship, as purification, as medicine—yes, that's grief as medicine. When our sadness is expressed, understood, and assimilated into the architecture of the spirit, we're one step closer to our authentic selves. Conversely, blunting or numbing the pain can impede our growth and send us spiraling further downward.

As a finger pointing to the moon, depression could be disguised instructions to forgive your husband, exercise five times a week, learn to love yourself, quit drinking, believe you did a good job caring for him as he was dying, be fearless in love, sleep eight hours a night, cry until all your tears are gone, dance your heart out, know that your husband does love you, resolve the trauma of the battlefield, restore your faith in your god, or stop eating all that ice cream and pie. Or any combination of the above, or many more. Depression is advice encrypted. It's not the enemy: it's information.

To take another example still, let's look at stress, a popular but vague word. When we think of antidotes for stress, we usually think of relaxation. That can certainly help: a good massage, a hot bath, or a day at the beach can reduce the boot prints of adrenaline and cortisol on our blood chemistry. But relaxation is not a solution. It's a byproduct of being complete and resolved. That may come about only when we change jobs, believe we're good enough, trust it will all work out, quit feeling victimized by our circumstances, know that we are loved, or stop having the affair. This means looking for the taproots of the stress, not at the frazzled nerves that are just its external, tangible form. Otherwise, the mere feeling of relaxation—whether induced with martinis, morphine, marijuana, or massage—might only delay our making tough, necessary choices. Behind stress, anxiety, and depression, we'll often find the reluctance to make hard decisions. We'll cover that in more detail in Chapter Five, "The Courage to Heal." It might help to remember that if a car on the highway is billowing clouds of smoke from the exhaust pipes, what it needs is not a smoke management program.

In Olivia's case, her adrenaline and cortisol had been in overdrive since those nights long ago in her grandfather's house. But focusing on only numbing their effects with tranquillizers would be like restraining the boy's hands holding the baseball bat—we'd still have an agitated boy. The patterns of stress were engraved onto her psyche and body during dark terrifying summer nights long ago.

If my patients' responses are a good measure, redefining our symptoms is easy. In part, it's similar to the lessons about the growth of human character we find in mythology and other literature and which I'll explore in Chapter Four, on health as transformation and medicine as catalyst. The idea that the challenges of living can help us strengthen character is a given. But what comes next takes the idea one step further, and may be surprising or even disorienting.

Appreciating symptoms

This next step, which may seem awkward or even unthinkable at first, is to appreciate the symptoms. When I suggest this to patients, they usually give me an awkward smile that's a combination of amusement, suspicions about my sanity, and then a recognition of its merits. The idea may sound comical, strange, or naïvely optimistic at first. But as one of my patients said, thoughtfully and gratefully, "This is a complete reversal of how we think of symptoms." It is. If the symptom's purpose is benevolent, if it's a wallop from the hands of the Earth's maternal wisdom, then honoring and appreciating it is good etiquette. As we might appreciate our friends and parents for their unwelcome though honest feedback, we can appreciate the symptom's good intentions even as we fidget under the pressure.

A symptom comes from the intelligence that informs the creation of the earth, stars, and galaxies, the trillions of biochemical events that occur in the human body, all life that has ever existed. These are impressive credentials for an experience we welcome as much as a dog barking at our heels. If that power is expressed in a human body as a headache or a back pain, then responding with gratitude and appreciation makes eminently good sense. In addition, doing so directly leads to reduced tension, which in turn helps in healing the symptom. Let's take all this even further and say we could respond to the symptom with reverence. If we can see the full existential backdrop of the symptom and find it in ourselves to revere the symptom, we do more than have a change of heart. We reposition ourselves in the politics of the natural world, being a collaborator with nature instead of a dissident.

To appreciate symptoms is to appreciate the wisdom in the physical and conscious universe present in every breath, every thought, every beat of the heart. The symptom is never just your personal possession. It also belongs to the entire universe.

Stress in relationships as a symptom

Another example of pain as a message is the distress of conflicts with friends and loved ones. Most of us know the misery of being angry with a spouse, intimate partner, or a family member. One of you may have humiliated the other at the family reunion. Back home, your eyes don't meet, your words are perfunctory, a coolness creeps into the house. Or you may be more overt by hurling spears of resentment back and forth across the kitchen table.

Regardless of its form, the disquiet that replaces an intimate serenity can be reinterpreted as a symptom. It's a symptom because it points at something else—the need for love and wholeness to be restored. Since the symptom's intention is always to elicit healing, then the disquiet, or that discomfort in the neck, chest, or belly, is the very incentive to forgive and make good. It will pursue us like a bloodhound until we end the conflict. That troubled feeling is love itself speaking, asking for its rightful place in your world, pressuring you to bring the sunlight back into your relationship with your loved ones.

We don't have much choice: if we don't heal the relationship, we're either a deflated balloon or a pair of restless legs.

As we look again beyond the emotional realm and consider the broader metaphysical implications, Jesuit priest and anthropologist Pierre Teilhard de Chardin helps us with these words:

> *Love is the internal, affectively apprehended aspect of the affinity which links and draws together the elements of the world, centre to centre... Love, in fact, is the expression and the agent of universal synthesis.*

He also wrote that we live in a conscious, intelligent universe that he called the *noosphere*. "Nous" is the ancient Greek root for mind, and noosphere is de Chardin's word for the entirety of the universe in which matter and consciousness are an integrated whole. Other writers have referred to similar ideas with words like omniverse and Kosmos—the latter being an ancient Greek word used to denote a conscious, divinely ordered universe. It's an idea we have already covered—that the universe is not only physical stuff, but a conscious ocean of wisdom. But Teilhard de Chardin's quote highlights an intriguing aspect of the idea: it's also more than just conscious or wise. He says, as do the mystics, that love is an integral part of the universe, blended like salt in the ocean's waters. It has a unifying, gravitational effect. It's a force drawing together earth, wind, fire, water, you and me.

Relationships demand resolution, without which we feel a tensile discomfort. This discomfort is like a wrestler pressing against us to restore wholeness in the relationship. It's an expression of de Chardin's idea that love is the affinity that draws together the fractured elements of the world—we can choose to heal the relationship or to worsen it. I don't mean to oversimplify the complexities of relationships, but in the end, it boils down to a simple choice: restore love or feel uneasy. Of course, the solution at times may be to compassionately end the relationship. As de Chardin would say, this push toward affinity is more than two minds and hearts yearning for union: it's the wisdom of the world itself seeking wholeness through two particular people.

When this wisdom insists, through the pain in our souls, that we resolve conflicts, we can appreciate the message instead of thinking it's a problem. In a similar way, many cancer survivors say they're grateful for how the illness enriched their lives: it helped them to appreciate just being alive, to love their friends and family more fully, and to learn to do what mattered most. The cancer journey shuffled their priorities to better reflect their authentic values. Loving their children and spending time with family became more important than earning money and most everything else.

Changing our defiance toward symptoms into gratitude and appreciation can help in two ways. The first is that being receptive to their good intentions feels better in itself. A benign attitude is in itself healthy and improves the chances of a better outcome. The second is that we might be more willing to take the symptom's counsel and act accordingly, whether it's going to see the doctor or changing lifestyle habits. By appreciating the symptom's role in our lives, we think more clearly and act more wisely. It's hard to understand something we hate.

Responding to symptoms

Given this perspective, then, how do we best respond to symptoms? How do we learn from them to thrive and flourish? A good start is to be curious about the symptom's intent and ask, "What's the message?", "What am I being asked to do?", "What's missing?", "What job is the symptom trying to get done?" By inquiring into the symptom's intentions, we then, as the ancient Chinese said, oblige the wisdom of heaven and earth. One message might be to see a doctor immediately, and, as always, you want to ensure that a seemingly harmless symptom is not signaling a hidden illness. Other messages can relate to virtually any area of our lives that needs to be changed. But regardless of the symptom, appreciation is a smart response when the brilliance of the omniverse, that august authority, comes knocking to speak personally with us. The pastor would have been better off had he respected the spiritual power behind the fire truck, boat, and helicopter.

While the message of some signs and symptoms will be easy to understand, others will be complex and may drive you to polish your skills as a health detective. Some symptoms will require professional help and thorough clinical consultations, but some will carry obvious messages, such as "Don't lift that refrigerator" or "Eat less cake." In any case, appreciating the logic behind symptoms is smart.

As another illustration, let's look at the common symptom of insomnia. Again, it's not a problem but a message. Difficulty in falling or staying asleep, while depressing or annoying, occurs for good reasons. The symptom may be asking you to drink less coffee and diet soda, or to be more optimistic about finding a job, or to forgive your husband or wife, or to exercise more, or to trust that your children will be all right on their first day at school. When you're awake at night, some part of you is hard at work solving a problem. Clearly, this part of you believes that fretting about the problem will help. So it's related to a need, and simply getting a massage, taking medications, or drinking herbal tea to relax doesn't get to that need. It may be asking us to eat healthily, or start exercising, or take electrolytes, or stop gnawing our nails about not having enough money.

Persuasion to flourish

A symptom persuades us to flourish. It's an injunction to become whole, fit, and strong. It asks that you evolve into the person your dog thinks you are.

With the world's wisdom expressed in so many ways—from azaleas blooming in the spring to headaches coming on in the fall—a symptom is just another of its voices, insisting on our constant growth and evolution. To see this, to see de Chardin's *affinity drawing all things in the world together*, is to penetrate the fog of the obvious. According to the ancient wisdom traditions, this affinity is grace, heaven's breath, animating the world and binding it together. Brian Swimme refers to this binding activity as allurement: a universal attraction of disparate parts seeking to come together in one whole. It is this allurement that de Chardin called love.

A symptom is more than a demand for the restoration of harmony. In the end, it's part of the sweeping arc of the world's power, persuading us, with either gentle or forceful hands, to shoot for the upper reaches of human possibility. Many symptoms are the result of being caught in the crossfire between our personal agendas and the one Mother Nature intends for us. With only a moment's reflection, it's clear who always wins. We may be obsessed with our goals, our health be damned, but this Mother doesn't care about our work and financial agendas: she only wants us to be healthy and whole. If we choose to remain seditious, she will find a way to stop us with one symptom or another. In her compassionate fierceness, she will shove us into bed with fatigue or aching joints or some other symptom, telling us to restore sanity and balance in our lives. Throughout, the allurement speaks. The Sufi poet Rumi wrote:

> *Don't turn your head. Keep looking*
> *at the bandaged place. That's where*
> *the light enters you.*
> > *And don't believe for a moment*
> *that you're healing yourself.*

Chapter Three

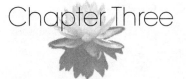

The Wellspring of Healing

A vast, profound, and prodigious impulse for healing and transformation lies within each of us. It's a self-organizing, evolutionary drive swirling about in body, mind, and soul. As the root of healing itself, it comes with the impressive provenance of having governed the mansion since life first appeared on the planet. Though the winds of healing come from within the body, mind, and soul, and though they have stunning powers, this idea is lost in the mayhem of our national conversation on health. It hasn't much influenced the reigning healthcare model, nor has it seeped into the street view of health.

In contrast, integrative medicine gives a starring role to the healing power inherent in the body. But it also nods to the strengths of other approaches to healing.

For most people I've seen in my practice, the idea that any improvement of their symptoms comes from within is news. I let them know the healing is theirs, not mine—I'm just the broker. With just a little reflection, it's evident enough, but this idea remains a blind spot in our culture. If patients become livelier and happier, I usually remind them that nothing is on those acupuncture needles, nothing was added, no medications were injected. The needles simply reorganized what was already in their bodies. On hearing that, they often look off into the distance and ponder for a few seconds. Then they look relieved and encouraged, sometimes smiling in recognition of an idea that makes great sense. On occasion, they protest and say no, you did it. But eventually, they come to accept and like the idea. I always enjoy seeing that look on their faces, as I trust it will change how they make decisions about their health for the rest of their lives.

On some occasions, though, they don't smile. As Cindy got off the treatment table after her first treatment, she was surprised to find herself serene and euphoric. She'd come to the session uneasy and muddled, with a long list of symptoms on her questionnaire. But now, she was wide-eyed and giddy as if on drugs. I then said that in a manner of speaking, she was the one who had done this: the euphoria had come from within her. The needles were agents, not the source. On hearing this, she sat down, absorbed the welcome news, and shed tears of relief.

Then there was Margaret, driving home on the highway after her first treatment. She was enjoying the deep relaxation she felt, but when she looked in the rearview mirror, she noticed a long line of cars backed up behind her. Puzzled at this unusual traffic configuration, she looked down and saw she was going forty miles an hour where the speed limit was fifty-five. She'd been driving at a speed that matched her sense of peace and calmness.

Poet Rainer Maria Rilke wrote, "Nowhere, Beloved, will world be but within us." In a similar vein, about 2,400 years earlier on the other side of the planet, Lao Tzu wrote that we can know the whole world by knowing what lies within us. Both Rilke and Lao Tzu point us inward, encouraging us to enter the worlds of mystery within. Similarly, in the search for health, we do well to go inward to the very wellspring of healing. More of the implications of this idea will be covered in Chapter Nine. But for now, I will focus on two facets of this idea.

One is the way it can help us make better decisions about our health. It can help us choose methods that support the intrinsic healing potential in mind and body, though there are times when stronger emergency measures are needed.

The other facet relates to the hope and optimism that the idea can evoke.

Many patients with persistent medical concerns are drenched in hopelessness. After dealing unsuccessfully with their symptoms or illnesses or from feeling weather-beaten by old age, pessimism is understandable. But when I tell them their bodies have extraordinary potential to heal, their eyes often brighten up. I'm not making a promise, as that's unethical in a clinical setting. But it's a balanced articulation of hope without promises, possibility without expectations, optimism without illusions. When I see the patient's eyes brighten on hearing this, it's easy to see how the idea is like fresh water on a dry garden.

To begin our exploration of the wellspring of healing, here's the story of Ann the painter.

Ann

In 2008, at the age of eighty-six, Ann resumed treatments with me after an absence of probably ten years or more. She's a soft, gentle but spirited soul with a quick, self-effacing sense of humor; we laugh often when she comes for her visits. In earlier years, she'd suffered from the shockwaves of her husband's alcoholism when he was still alive. In the last several years, she'd been distraught by her son's madcap alcoholic life. Throughout most of her life, she'd kept her chin up. But when her son went broke and became homeless, the strain was overwhelming. In June of 2008, after a couple of years of this stress, Ann was diagnosed with stage IV small-cell lung cancer. By the time her doctors diagnosed her, it had already metastasized from her right lung to her ribs, spine, right hip, and many lymph nodes. About half of it was in her bones. With a diagnosis of a stage IV cancer, it was time, as the euphemism goes, to put her affairs in order. As Ann thought about the effect of the stress about her son might have had, she said, "If stress can cause cancer, that did it." Her oncologist said that with chemotherapy, she might have a year to live.

Without it, six months.

Throughout her life, Ann had taken good care of her body. She had stopped smoking forty-six years earlier. She ate plenty of grains, fresh fruit, and vegetables. She meditated and prayed. She led a peaceful life painting in her studio by the river. No one in her family had gotten cancer. So the news was shocking.

Ann had recently fallen in love with a man of about the same age. Whenever she spoke of her new sweetheart, as she called him, her face lit up. As the English say, she was besotted. After being a widow for decades, getting into a romantic relationship was an unexpected turn of events. Now at eighty-six, she found herself intensely in love with her soul mate. She laughed as she noted the quirky timing of the fates.

As we started her treatments, I suggested she receive acupuncture once or twice weekly. This would not be treatment for cancer, but would instead give her the support to stay as strong and energetic as possible. If her body could become more energetic and resilient, she might get through her chemotherapy more easily and she might feel better emotionally. As research has suggested, the acupuncture might reduce side effects of chemotherapy like nausea and fatigue. After I recommended that she use other natural healing methods as well, she set out on a regimen of nutritional supplements recommended by a naturopath, a very healthy diet, journaling, meditation, hypnotherapy, massage, and acupressure. During our visits, we spoke about how she might find some semblance of peace even with dire prospects on the near horizon—regardless of what might happen with her body, regardless of any diagnosis at all. Whether she lived or died, whether she was sick or not, a peaceful heart was worthwhile. She recognized that if she were to die, which seemed inevitable, she wanted to do so with a calm heart.

During her visits, Ann and I spent much time talking about finding this peace, about learning to breathe easy about her circumstances of the past, present, or future. Easier said than done with the eyes of death glaring at her, but perhaps possible. In my view, we were working toward what all of us need anyway, whether we have five weeks or fifty years left on the planet. The nearness of death just lends an urgency to get the work done faster.

Before long, Ann came to feel resolved. Although she was saddened at the thought of her impending death, she took solace in having lived a fulfilling life. She saw that her diagnosis was not a tragedy. After all, she'd lived longer than she'd expected, and since she had to go sooner or later, she became grateful for the life she'd been given, for just being alive in the moment. With a true acceptance of her son's disordered life and of its inevitability, she learned, in her words, to detach with love. Echoing the words of Alcoholics Anonymous and Al-Anon, she said she had let go and let God.

It's noteworthy that CAM (complementary and alternative medicine) methods, just like meaningful conversations of this sort, can be helpful whether we're sick or not. This differentiates them strategically from the usual approaches to the treatment of disease. They're intended to increase energy, vitality, and awareness—regardless of whether a person is healthy or unwell, whether she is symptomatic or not. They're not intended to treat disease but to balance, revitalize, and rejuvenate people with any kind of symptom at any

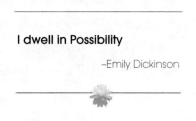

I dwell in Possibility

–Emily Dickinson

stage of health. When combined with chemotherapy, surgery, or radiation, they might improve the odds and provide some relief from the side effects of the chemotherapy. The general public sometimes misperceives CAM methods to be an alternative to conventional medicine, and while that's true in some cases, they can almost always be a complement.

So Ann began her cancer journey: an integrative approach using chemotherapy as well as a full array of natural healing methods. From her oncologist, she received several rounds of chemotherapy plus a bone-building medication that has been shown in some cases to be helpful in treating bone cancers.

Then after a few months, unexpectedly, the fates again intervened. But not in the way everyone had anticipated. In October 2008, just five months after her diagnosis, Ann's oncologist told her that the cancer had essentially vanished. The only remnant was the original tumor in her right lung, but it had shrunk dramatically to 1.1 centimeters and was inactive. The cancer in the bones was gone, the lymph nodes clear. The scans showed no signs of cancer anywhere else.

No one had dared talk remission: not I, her oncologist, her other healthcare providers, nor Ann herself. In a long discussion later, Ann's oncologist told me that she'd hoped the chemotherapy would give Ann a few months, not a new lease on life, and that she'd never seen anything like this in her long career. The chances of survival had been nil.

The intention of the integrative therapies like acupuncture and massage had been to support Ann's overall vitality and resilience, not to target the cancer cells. We were all astounded. Ann was ecstatic from the mystifying but wonderful news. Today, at the age of eighty-nine, she's still madly in love with her sweetheart and comes for a tune-up treatment with me once a month.

I tell this story as one illustration of that mysterious but compelling healing potential that lives and breathes in all of us. It's the deep well of healing, of possibility, that's already and always within. It might be active, or sitting dormant behind a wailing wall of ailments, but whatever expressed itself in Ann's healing is available to all of us. This doesn't at all suggest that results like hers are commonplace or to be expected from an integrative approach to cancer. Her story simply hints at the possibility within the human body.

This healing power comes from a body informed by the wisdom of the universe, by angels with muscle, cherubs with medical training, minor gods of the clinic. According to the ancient traditions, this wisdom, which is power, is the creative principle of life itself. It speaks through the wind and the sun, the waters and the earth, all animals big and small, and is found in the farthest winds of the universe.

It's not a merely biological force, but part of Swimme's idea of allurement, a basic power of the universe, a magnetic affection that the different pieces of the universe have for each other. Whether it shows up as two people falling in love, the healing of a wound, the growth of a metropolis, the magnetism between galaxies, or an apple falling off a tree onto a man's head, it's an integrative force that informs the physical and conscious universe. The wellspring of healing is life seeking itself, always in motion, shaping itself out of the void, pushing for communion within and between us. When we heal and flourish, it's this force, this *élan vital*, coming through the individual aperture called "you."

In recent decades, researchers have succeeded in mapping the whole human genome. This, understandably, has led to excitement about potential breakthroughs in clinical applications. With the blueprints of health and disease now at our disposal, scientists tell us that this will steer medical and pharmaceutical research in promising new directions over the coming decades. That is encouraging news.

But genes are not the source of healing. They are parts of the machine; they help explain the architecture of disease and health. On the other hand, the wellspring of healing—the source of change itself—is the invisible milieu that gave birth to genes in the first place. Genes are machine parts, not the manufacturer nor the architect. They are the software program, not the programmer.

None of us involved in Ann's care can explain what happened. Did the chemotherapy alone produce this change against all odds and expectations? Possibly. But, as the oncologist said, the odds were as close to zero as they could get. Was it then the combination of chemotherapy and the CAM treatments? Possibly. But then again, some research has shown that about two percent of cancer patients will heal from their cancer anyway. For a senior in her late eighties, with end-stage cancer, the odds were most likely far slimmer than two percent. So the outcome was not impossibly beyond the razor-thin probabilities. But even if it had fallen within that tiny range of probabilities, the idea of spontaneous remission is a description, not an explanation.

This much we can safely infer: *the human body has transformative abilities at every moment, at virtually any age.* Whether through natural methods only or through a combination of conventional and natural methods, the body can engage the engines of healing and elicit the powers of wholeness. The healing powers of the world are at work whether what disappears is a simple headache or stage IV lung cancer.

In the last hundred years, this self-organizing power to heal has been thrust into the shadows by technology's dazzling lights. But prior to that, and to this day, the traditions of the ancients, including those of the Native American, Inuit, Tibetan, Indian, Greek, and Chinese, assert that the origins of this power were the Great Spirit, or Mother Earth and Father Sky, or Shiva and Shakti, or Aesclepius and his daughters Hygea, Panacea, Iaso, Aseso, Aegleia, or other celestial icons—not to be tossed in the corner just because their names are metaphors.

We've lost faith in the pure and simple ways of the earth and sky. Because the ethos of nature is under our noses at all times, we don't notice it, just as we forget the comfortable old shirt we wore all day. We are unimpressed with the curious magic of eating plants, leaves, roots, fish, and chickens only to have them converted into our skin and teeth, arms and legs, eyes and ears. We don't notice that our bodies are true alchemists that use the input of beans, carrots, beef, eggs, and potatoes and then, to borrow a word from *Calvin and Hobbes*, transmogrify them into the output of a body that walks and talks, that knows just how much oxygen to inhale, that neutralizes stress hormones while we sleep, that reads spreadsheets, dances the rhumba, rides bikes, and makes the heart beat about four billion times during its career. By remembering the impossibly miraculous nature of the body, we can deepen our trust in the wellspring of healing. It exists in every cell of our bodies. We are walking miracles.

The awareness of this miraculous force was perhaps what Rilke encouraged when he wrote, "*Truly* being here is glorious." For some people, realizing this comes from a spiritual experience, whether spontaneous or cultivated. For others, it comes after a close encounter with death: a stroke, brain aneurysm, or a near-death experience that took them beyond the last precipice of life and back. In these cases, people often speak of a sparkling new awareness of the beauty and preciousness of life.

Truly being here, *just* being here, was more than enough for Ann, who said, "It gave me so much joy and gratitude for being alive. Every day is a celebration." As people feel this meaningfulness in their hearts, they see the world with new eyes. They come to appreciate the wonders formerly disguised as the prosaic: one's own breath, just being alive, the morning sun, a good cup of coffee, the husband or wife they'd taken for granted, annoying children who instantly become things of blinding beauty. As the frenetic, crazy-making pace of contemporary life distracts us and amplifies the volume of the picayune and the irrelevant, it often takes tragedy to remind us of what's essential.

Although the inherent power of the body, mind, and soul to heal themselves usually goes unnoticed, it ought to leave us speechless. As it deserves far more time at center stage, I spend a good deal of my time in the treatment room explaining this idea to my patients. And it's more than another good idea; rather, it's a singular way of looking at the essence and the nature of healing— with massive implications for our lives. What holds the reins is the old model, in which we are accustomed to letting an external agent like a medication fix a problem. Again, there are plenty of conditions that must be controlled with medications, and medications have provided millions with a better life or life itself. But when the ways of the old model are applied indiscriminately, we might misplace both the opportunity to heal from within. If the inherent healing potential of mind and body became a philosophical cornerstone for our healthcare system, we would see revolutionary advances come about.

In the first chapter, I pointed out that the body is not a thing, but a suggestion of deeper truths. It's a 3D representation of intangibles, a potentiality, not just a collection of flesh and bones. It's a verb, not a noun; or, as the ancients put it, the body is energy. Deepak Chopra, M.D., and others have written extensively about the idea that our bodies are pure energy, pure potentiality. We are not only physical chunks of biological stuff, but bundled energy, an aggregation of possibilities. In rethinking the very paradigms of health, these sorts of ideas— the ethereal, abstract principles—are not just exercises in imagination. They can lead to big, concrete effects.

The practical effects of galvanizing this healing potential are many. For one, you're more likely to feel responsible for your health. By understanding that you're affecting your health and your symptoms by what you do, all day every day, you might make wiser choices. For another, you'll be more likely to stop fixing just the symptoms and to dig deeper under the soil toward the roots of optimal vitality. No side effects occur when the body heals from within. When calling upon Nature to reorganize itself in harmony with its original schematics, it's not possible to have side effects. Healing aggravations, such as the purging of toxins from the body, or the catharsis of unfinished emotional business, can certainly occur. But those are not side effects. Instead, they're the essence of healing in action. They're the necessary purging of the detritus hidden in either the psyche or the body.

As described in Chapter Two, healing is more than an individual physical event. To think of "my" healing or "my" body is grammatically and socially correct, but philosophically imprecise. We can, instead, remember that what runs through our veins is not of our own creation but part of a grander universal design and that the illusion of being isolated from the rest of the world is just that: *maya*, a fantasy, a trick. When PMS, a headache, or a back pain improve, the whole world is healing itself at a particular location called you. When Ramana Maharshi said, "Whereas, that which is, is only spiritual," he was including the human body and its healing potential.

Three types of treatment approaches

Next, here are a few distinctions that may be helpful as we explore the nature of healing. We can divide all clinical actions into three broad categories, each with different strategies and effects:

- Control
- Substitute
- Catalyze

Control. Controlling methods are those used by a health professional to take command of a medical condition that is dangerous, chaotic, and unlikely to correct itself. In these circumstances, the damage is so severe that the body can't heal itself or restore order on its own. These conditions are usually found in emergency rooms or intensive care units, and include gunshot wounds, broken bones, trauma from a car accident, pneumonia, arterial bleeding, and severe viral or bacterial infections. Since the conditions won't correct themselves, the doctors, nurses, and other staff members must aggressively manipulate bones, breath, blood, brain, or heart to keep the patient alive. The methods for controlling include surgery, CPR, defibrillators, blood transfusions, organ transplants, massive infusions of antibiotics, steroids, narcotics, and so on. They are manipulation and control in the finest sense.

Beyond the emergency room, many other conditions require the controlling, aggressive use of medications such as those necessary for preventing seizures, the rejection of transplanted organs, the chaos of uncontrolled psychosis, the degeneration of multiple sclerosis. The medications and the machines wrestle with pathological drives to subdue them. Thankfully, that kind of control and domination has saved millions of lives. And this is where conventional medicine is unparalleled. Psychiatrist and acupuncturist Michael Smith, M.D., who was founder and director of the South Bronx's Lincoln Hospital Recovery Center which treated about two hundred drug addicts with acupuncture daily for four decades, says that when a patient is hanging off the edge of a cliff by his fingers, it's not the time to ask if he's been taking his vitamins, getting enough sleep, and eating his vegetables. We can focus on wellness later. Controlling methods pull people off the cliff edge, when survival is the main goal.

Substitute. At other times, we use substitutes for what the body might do for itself. The most common of substitutes is medication. Under normal circumstances, we're capable of producing the hormones, enzymes, and the many types of natural pharmaceuticals that keep us ticking. We have our own internal pharmacy, ready to release all the natural substances that keep the body humming.

We can ward off inflammation, infection, and cell degeneration with endogenous stuff brought forth by actions like a rigorous exercise regimen, natural foods, deep rest, and a calm heart. But when, for example, inflammation creates pain, we're accustomed to substitute for the body's own anti-inflammatory functions by taking medications like ibuprofen. If our immune system is weak, we might compensate for its deficient antihistamine production by taking over-the-counter remedies or prescription medications.

If we haven't been producing enough serotonin for maintaining our good moods, then we might take anti-depressants to substitute for our brain's own muscle for producing the substance.

At times, a substitute is a godsend. In serious or overwhelming circumstances, it's appropriate and necessary. But the disadvantage is that we might block the inherent potential to heal if, in the long run, we use medications to substitute for the hard work needed to keep ourselves healthy, if we use them in place of the discipline needed to eat well, exercise, and to make the tough choice of trading off a few indulgences for what's healthy. The potential for healing is reduced because substitutes treat the symptom, not the roots. They shoot the messenger, or at least tie him up and toss him into a corner. Substitutes often ignore the reasons why the symptom came about in the first place. This is similar to someone turning off the smoke alarm buzzing in the night and then going back to bed.

Whether the diagnosis is high blood pressure, anxiety, or painful joints, we can, in many cases, meet the body's needs with natural methods. Of course, preventing illnesses is far easier than correcting them after the fact. But to a good extent, we already have the medications we need right here in the ecology of our homegrown bodies. Whole foods, a good exercise regimen, and zest in the psyche keep the shelves of the internal pharmacy well stocked.

Our culture, unfortunately, has also had the predilection for another type of substitute. A high dosage of donuts, cake, cookies, or ice cream will help us feel less aggravated about office politics or the boss's illogical decisions. This big bolus of sugar and fat literally produces a pharmacological effect in our bodies. Five cups of coffee to jump-start the day can substitute for the rest and exercise that lead to a natural flow of energy. Beer, wine, or liquor can sedate frayed nerves or substitute for the boldness we need to address a problem head on. Alcohol might provide momentary self-confidence that would be better nurtured through self-understanding and reflection. Instead of keeping the situation in perspective, or communicating effectively, or otherwise solving problems, we can create a false sense of wellbeing through alcohol, drugs, or the abuse of prescription drugs. Other substitutes include hypersexuality, overspending, an obsession with appearances, an addiction to overwork, or a compulsion to take care of everyone but ourselves. We're limited only by our imagination in creating substitutes.

Unfortunately, these are all band-aids with potentially unhealthy effects. They don't lead to authentic wellbeing. While substitutes do make us feel better, the good feelings are only caricatures. In the long run, we risk becoming increasingly dependent on them, whether they're anti-depressants or alcohol, pot or pastries. On the other hand, the glow of a good laugh over dinner with friends, or the flush of wellbeing from a long swim, or the luminosity of having a child snuggled in your arms are all measures of authentic vitality.

When trying to choose from a number of healthcare options, ask yourself if the method is a substitute for what your body might do for itself. The decision may need to be made with the advice of a health professional, but at least consider if you can create the desired improvement through a lifestyle change.

As an example, let's look at the widespread complaint of anxiety. Reviewing what we've seen so far, anxiety is a symptom. A symptom is a message, not a problem. Next, it's a signal coming from the intrinsic healing potential in the mind and body. So instead of flailing at the windmill of anxiety or dulling its edges with natural or pharmaceutical substitutes, we can ask, "What gem of an insight is my anxiety trying to give me?" If we can answer that question, then we're closer to the nucleus. The anxiety may contain any number of messages, like relax, you'll survive if you get laid off. Or it's OK, he does love you. Or stop the caffeine and alcohol. Or let go of your grief and guilt because it's time to move on. Or exercise for a half-hour five times a week. Or don't try to control everything.

A symptom such as anxiety is a roadmap, however vague, leading to the real "cure." But if we don't trust the body-mind's ability to correct itself, we readily turn to substitutes. Whether we use whiskey, massage, acupuncture, herbs, or sleeping medications, we may be avoiding the necessary changes.

A young patient of mine who worked for a federal agency knew that his bouts of severe diarrhea and weight loss were triggered by stress. While he'd been treated with medications for the clearly identified medical condition of ulcerative colitis, he nevertheless noticed that when major life stresses came his way, he was prone to get worried and pessimistic—and that's exactly when his symptoms were provoked. After he and I talked about symptoms as educators, I asked him what he thought their message might be. Without a moment's hesitation, he said they were telling him, "Suck it up, big guy." He knew that in addition to the physical aspects of his illness, a psychological and spiritual imperative was being issued. He knew he needed to learn to be courageous and rise above his resignation and passivity. The presence of his symptoms was an audition. The risk, then, was that the use of medications, though necessary for now, might distract him from the need to awaken his inner tiger.

Catalyze. The third type of clinical action is one that catalyzes inherent healing potential. A catalytic method's purpose is to strengthen your ability to heal from the bottom up, to arouse dormant possibilities, to arouse the sleeping dragon. It opens the sluices of the wellspring of healing. It brings forth possibility, stirring the sleepy but benevolent demigods of healing.

Just as water, fertilizer, soil, and sunlight catalyze the growth of cilantro and roses, a catalytic method evokes the coherence needed for vitality in the human body. But a gardener doesn't create roses or cilantro. She seduces them into existence. Similarly, a catalytic approach to health allows the latencies of the human body to flower.

The body holds extraordinary promise, a transformative tonic that in

other venues will turn an infant in diapers into the president of the United
States and a small seed into a 275-foot redwood tree with a base diameter
of thirty-six feet. We can trust this promise coiled in the spine of human
possibility to help us shape-shift into something unpredictably new. We may
not be able to forecast where it will take us, but it's a strapping possibility
within. The entire next chapter will be devoted to how we can catalyze growth
and transformation.

Catalytic methods include naturopathy, massage, yoga, tai chi, nutrition
counseling, exercise, acupuncture, homeopathy, Ayurveda, herbs, herbal
medicine, natural supplements, chiropractic, osteopathic manipulative
treatment, speech therapy, psychotherapy, music therapy, guided imagery,
Reiki, coaching, meditation, breathwork, spiritual practices, and more. Some
are ancient, some new, but they all galvanize your strengths into a healthier
you. When you feel euphoric after a massage, it's because the potential for
euphoria had been waiting for you. The same is true whenever people feel
fresh and awake from any of these catalytic methods. The practitioner doesn't
create serenity, elation, or liveliness. She extracts them as she might gold from
a mine. In a culture habituated to evoking pleasure with external stimuli, it's
easy to forget how much aliveness lies sleeping within.

Comparisons of the three approaches

Each of the three types of methods—controlling, substitutive, and catalytic—
has its strengths, limitations, and best uses. Knowing the differences between
them can help you choose sensibly. For example, any type of emergency
situation, such as a stroke, heart attack, kidney failure, or pneumonia, needs
a controlling intervention. The same goes for serious chronic diseases such
as cancer, congestive heart failure, cirrhosis of the liver, or advanced diabetes.
The risks of death or serious disability are high, and the conditions will career

downhill unless controlled. Fortunately, many people can intuitively sense when they need a controlling method. If my patients have a medical crisis, they never call me but go straight to the emergency room.

As for the limitations of controlling methods, they clearly don't promote wellness and optimal vitality. But that's not their intention. They're designed to pull people off the cliff's edge.

Substitutive methods are often necessary when the body is unable to restore order on its own. Sometimes a fine line separates a substitutive method from a controlling one. Severe pains, infections, or other diseases such as diabetes may call for a high dose of medications—which are generally substitutive. But in these circumstances, they are, in effect, controlling methods. In severe depression, patients can get themselves off the cliff edge with anti-depressants, the better to work later on the depression's roots.

But for millions of people, medications are substitutes for the often-laborious work of caring well for the mind and body. This predilection for substitutes feeds our healthcare crisis. If public policy better encouraged prevention and catalytic approaches to health, we'd have far fewer illnesses in the first place. After years of neglecting the simplest needs of the human body, substitutions and controls become necessary for many of us. But these are costly in time, not just in dollars. They often perpetuate the cycle of neglect if the unhealthy behavior isn't reversed. With a healthy diet, exercise, and a balanced lifestyle, we can catalyze health and forego many medications and medical procedures. Again, scientists estimate that this applies to more than 75 percentof chronic diseases.

Catalytic methods elicit human potential. They start by being collaborative with symptoms and then helping patients transform their lives from the ground up. They take up where conventional medicine stops, helping patients go from the absence of disease to feeling great. Controlling or substitutive methods can't do this, but then again, that's not their purpose.

Another difference between the three methods is the speed of change. In addition to being powerful, the controlling methods work fast. A tumor can be removed in only a few hours. Substitutive methods such as medications can also work quickly, kicking in within minutes, although many of them can take days and weeks to exert their influence. Catalytic methods, while they also may work fast at times, often work more slowly, just as getting in shape at the gym takes time. Gently nudging a person toward health can take months or years.

The problems of substitution

As we've seen, one drawback to substitutive methods is that they don't get to the roots of the problem. If we take anti-inflammatories for pains that would otherwise clear up with exercise, diet, and lifestyle changes, we may be pulling ourselves into a downward spiral. Allergy medications are another example of substitutes. A clean, whole-foods diet, a vigorous exercise regimen, and a low-stress lifestyle can strengthen the immune system and reduce or eliminate some allergies. But substitutes are tempting, and often irresistible, because they're quick, convenient, and usually covered by insurance. That can dampen our incentive to make the tough choice to change our unhealthy habits. In place of exercising four or five times a week and taking the time to cook healthy meals with fresh whole foods, it's easier to pop a substitute into our mouths in a second.

In summary, controlling methods pull us off the brink of death or disaster. Substitutive methods help us manage and survive. Catalytic methods help us flourish. Since the three can overlap, an integrative approach to medicine uses all of them as necessary. The challenge for each person is to find the best combination of methods.

The implications of the three approaches in our healthcare system are enormous. Great reductions in cost would be realized from the widespread use of catalytic approaches to health—approaches that would evoke the strength, resilience, and integrity that already live in the temple of the body and mind. This would prevent a horde of illnesses, eliminating millions of prescriptions and surgeries. Catalytic methods can not only lower the risk of getting sick in the first place; they can improve outcomes of surgery and medication, reduce the number of hospitalizations, and can often be used in place of substitutes like medications. Translating this potential into sweeping policy changes and economic restructuring in our healthcare system is another matter entirely. But understanding these principles is a start.

It may be just around the corner

A couple of patient stories will highlight how catalytic methods, which are often slow to work, can sometimes work quickly. I hesitate to tell stories of quick results because they're not the norm and can raise expectations too high. Usually, I urge patients to expect a slow pace of improvements while they heal naturally. But occasionally, a breakthrough is just around the corner.

James was a stocky, thirty-eight-year-old, rugby-playing Irishman whose quiet ways contrasted with his solid physique. He had come to see me for allergies and sinusitis, with the symptoms of sneezing, a runny nose, and watery eyes. He was miserable. When I asked him when this first started, he said it had plagued him nonstop since he was three years old in Ireland. During his first visit, I suggested that he stop using dairy products to see if he was lactose intolerant. Since he drank a lot of milk, it was worth a test. After a two-week test period, he could then resume his dairy intake and see how he reacted. He agreed to do this, and I gave him his first acupuncture treatment. When he returned the following week, he said that his allergies, sinusitis, and all his symptoms had vanished completely. I can't say how much of the change was due to the dietary changes and how much to the acupuncture. But thirty-five years of serious sinusitis had disappeared overnight.

In a similar case, Kendra was a thirty-year-old executive who came to me feeling unwell. Tall, athletic, smart, and attractive, she'd gone far in the corporate world in a short time. But since moving from the U.S. to the dark winter of a near-Arctic climate in Europe, she'd been tired and blue. She thought this might be due to a combination of culture shock, the long distance from friends and family, and the unrelenting darkness. Her symptoms, which she'd had before, included irritable bowel syndrome, stomach pains, bloating, and swelling in her joints, all of which had gotten worse after moving across the Atlantic. She also spoke about her loneliness, anger, sense of abandonment, and some of the emotional struggles of her childhood. But I suspected, after reviewing her health questionnaire and completing the examination, that she might have an intolerance to gluten, a protein found in wheat, barley, rye, and spelt. Gluten intolerance has become more common in the U.S. during the last couple of decades, so I now suggest to many patients that they test for it by going on a gluten-free diet for a week or two.

When Kendra came back several days later for her second visit, she looked entirely different. She was glowing, her voice was vibrant, and you could see a new glint in her eyes. The tiredness, moodiness, stomach pains, and bloating had disappeared from one acupuncture treatment and a gluten-free diet. As with James, I couldn't tell how much of change came from the treatment and how much from the absence of offending foods. There would be more work for Kendra to do, and since she was returning to Europe, I wasn't sure how long the changes would last. But a door had opened.

Few conditions are this simple to eliminate. But on the other hand, many stubborn symptoms may not be as entrenched as they appear. The key point is that a catalytic method and the removal of dietary antagonists helped James and Kendra eradicate months and years of distress that substitutive methods hadn't touched. The healing potential waiting in their bodies needed only a nudge to come forth and change their lives.

Persistence

The impulse for healing is remarkably persistent. Throughout the difficult times we all must face eventually, it helps to remember that this innate healing potential is a sturdy, reliable ally. Even when all seems lost, it still waits—loyal, ready, stalwart—and is ready to surprise us. Even under the clouds of neglect and poor health, the durable human body is ready to recast itself in new form. Given the noxious diets and the sedentary, pressured lifestyles of many people, it's remarkable that we're not sicker.

The wellspring of healing is a self-generating, renewable resource. While the idea can help any of us feel more optimistic, it's especially relevant to seniors, who, as they get older and feel the creakiness of aging, often conclude prematurely that it's all downhill from here on.

I'm struck that so many people describe the effects of aging with the exact words, "I'm falling apart." Perhaps they have a subconscious understanding of health as integration and illness as dis-integration. Perhaps it's just due to its popularity as idiom. But I've seen countless people resuscitate, resurrect, and revitalize after they'd claimed the end was near. Over months or years, they might have been getting weaker—their life force evaporating, their horizons shrinking, their breath withering. As the bleakness of death approached, all the controlling medications, substitutive therapies, and catalytic methods were a pittance. Sometimes the patients were so fragile that I'd worry about a heart attack or stroke waiting just around the corner. But then, maybe through a combination of human intervention and the fates, they'd revive and live for many more years. From seeing this repeatedly over the years, my trust in the tenacity of the life force has been greatly strengthened. Healing potential is one stubborn mule. It's available to us in most circumstances, whether we're young or old. I'll illustrate with a story about Julie. Although she was young, her story still points to this tenacity.

When Julie first came to see me years ago, she was an account executive in her early thirties who had suffered from the effects of cocaine and alcohol abuse. She was also an admitted workaholic. She had tried rehab, psychotherapy, Alcoholics Anonymous, and Narcotics Anonymous, but her health was still sliding downhill, the addictions firmly entrenched. Though she got drunk and high on cocaine several times a week, she still managed to function at work.

Over the first few months of acupuncture, she would feel relaxed and rejuvenated from each treatment, but I never felt that we were making any appreciable progress. Our work seemed as progressive as turning a light switch on and off. Though I made participation in AA or NA a necessary condition for her to receive acupuncture, her attendance at the meetings eventually became erratic. Nevertheless, over the course of a year, she started showing small signs of improvement. This included a drop in her cocaine use, and then, half a year later, the end of her habit. But she continued working sixty and seventy hours a week.

When Julie stopped using cocaine, she started drinking more. No matter how much acupuncture she received, no matter how much I counseled her, and no matter how many AA meetings she attended, she did what she wanted. She was a train on her own tracks and continued to charge headfirst into her destructive habits. But she loved acupuncture and assured me she was changing. She insisted on continuing with the treatments despite my doubts as to its usefulness for her.

Then one year she quit her job and started her own company. This meant working ninety to a hundred and twenty hours a week, sometimes from six in the morning to midnight, seven days a week, months on end. To counteract the stress and to relax, she drank a six-pack or two every night. All the usual health concerns—nutrition, exercise, rest, adequate sleep, and so on—were tossed out like a tattered doll. She felt she couldn't relax for a moment because her employees depended on the company for their livelihood.

This dreadful cycle went on for years. During this period, Julie rarely made the changes to which she'd agreed, even simple ones like drinking more water, going to an AA meeting, cutting back her hours, or eating a healthy meal once in a while instead of burgers and fries. They were all ignored. Because she was using acupuncture to substitute for tough choices, we were going nowhere. So one day I told her that in good conscience, I couldn't continue treating her. I felt this was necessary since I'd been colluding with her inertia and the patterns of addiction. The treatments had offset the effects of a harsh lifestyle and alcohol abuse, enabling her to continue with destructive habits. I had let her use the catalytic method of acupuncture as a substitute for hard decisions. After a long conversation, she understood that she'd been hiding behind the acupuncture.

I again said that I would treat her only if she implemented some healthy changes in her lifestyle and if she attended a minimum of one AA meeting a week, no matter how swollen her work hours.

As the years went by, she would come several months at a time for a burst of treatments, then disappear into her work again. In the meantime, she rushed headlong into the stresses of learning leadership skills and business savvy, ever on the run. But the business grew, and after the company eventually became solvent, she made time for nurturing her health.

Then she entered a rocky relationship with a man who also was an alcoholic. When she saw her destructive behavior mirrored in him, she started to drink less. Almost imperceptibly, year after year, she became more consistent in taking care of herself.

Today, her company is thriving and earns millions. She has a couple of drinks on occasion, despite knowing that the AA standard is that not a drop of alcohol should cross her lips. But she nevertheless has gotten healthier by resting more, sleeping more, exercising a little, and eating more whole foods.

She has turned the corner, and I feel reassured, for the first time, that she has made it to solid ground. Her eyes are clearer and softer now. All this took nine years.

I marvel at the coiled energy of her life, that uncompromising resolve hidden in the cells of her body. As we've seen, this force, this resolve, is more than Julie's personal entitlement: it's the same force that gives birth to trillions of animals, plants, and trees, and to billions of babies—the creative force of life itself. What worked in Julie works in all of us, waiting, breathing, present, possible.

Potential in our later years

This hardiness of the life force is especially relevant to the elderly. They, and even those in their forties and fifties, often attribute their symptoms or illnesses to aging. They usually assume that their aches and pains are irreversible. While that may be true in many cases, even then it's worth being receptive to unforeseen possibilities. It may not all be as ominous as it seems.

First, it helps to remember that chronological and biological aging are different. One is a measure, like a yardstick. The other is a physiological change. Inches, feet, and yards don't exist, nor do calendar days and months: they're measures. While aging by the calendar certainly leads to cellular aging, and while we can't control the passage of time, we can apply footbrakes to biological aging. Study after study has shown that people who exercise regularly are healthier and happier than their counterparts who stay on the couch. They also tend to live longer. In some studies, people in their seventies who exercised rigorously looked about twenty years younger than their peers who did little or no exercise. We can not only put the brakes on aging, we can even reverse it up to a point.

To illustrate the difference between aging by the calendar and aging physically, here's an analogy. Imagine bringing home two bunches of grapes from the grocery store, then putting one on the back porch in the hot sun and the other in the fridge. A week later when you compare the two, the grapes in the fridge will be firm and fresh, while those on the porch will be rotten. They're both the same "age," so how do we explain the entirely different conditions? They're at entirely different biological ages.

The way we normally think of aging is inaccurate. It's more accurate to say one bunch of grapes was biologically healthy and the other wasn't. That's more relevant than the number of days they've aged as we determine their health. The conditions that led to either freshness or deterioration determined the results, not the number of days. Similarly, that's how we can view the nature of aging. We wouldn't think of saying that 1,250 feet is the cause of the Empire State Building's height, but that's similar to the logic of saying our chronological age causes illness. The achiness and creakiness we attribute to aging come from the deterioration of biological processes in the body, not to this yardstick we call time. Since aging over time does parallel biological deterioration, there's obviously a limit to how much we can slow or reverse the effects of aging. But, on the whole, seniors have far more potential to heal than they think.

Arthritis is arthritis—young people can have it and many seniors don't. So it can't be caused by aging, even though aging predisposes us to it. A sore, stiff body can often be revitalized by the right exercise, diet, and infusions of love and joy into the soul. It helps to keep in mind that we can heal at any age.

Many seventy-five-year-olds are sprightly and fit, while many thirty-year-olds are rusty and flaccid beyond their years. Old age is an idea, a concept, while the deterioration of cellular function, tissues, and organs is a physical event. This deterioration is due in part to oxidation, which, in brief, is the loss of electrons from atoms. This is what happens to a grape left in the sun. When a car rusts or a tree rots, that's also oxidation. In recent years, research has suggested that oxidation can be reduced through nutrition, exercise, and the right supplements. The increased popularity of antioxidant supplements such as turmeric, grape seed extract, ginger, green tea extract, and resveratrol is an outgrowth of this research. Fruits and vegetables have strong antioxidant effects.

Though we can't turn back the clock, we can scrub off some of the rust of oxidation. Studies have shown that people even in their eighties can reduce their biological ages through exercise and a diet of whole foods. In addition, other research has suggested that living with a strong social network and pursuing a fulfilling spiritual life are important for our health and longevity.

Many of my elderly patients come to me resigned to a gray future, so I spend a good amount of time encouraging them to remember the bulldog tenacity of the healing potential that still resides in their flesh and bones. For most seniors, rejuvenation is still possible. But a mood of resignation to the tides of aging is itself another problem to be addressed. If they believe they can't be healthier, they've already reduced the odds. The challenge, for patients of any age, is not necessarily pessimism, but the blinders on the imagination imposed by the stridency of pain or exhaustion, by the myth that they can't rejuvenate at their age.

While clinicians can't offer guarantees, it helps both the patient and clinician to at least consider if some of the complaints of old age might be reversed or reduced. It's more philosophically honest to have an inquiring mind than to start by concluding that progress is impossible. Why not test the hypothesis that you can get healthier regardless of your age? When the question of "What's possible?" is turned into a lens through which we imagine the future, we can see more than we might through the lens of "I'm too old to become healthier."

The story of Rick, a seventy-seven-year-old retiree with back pain, illustrates this point. After a few acupuncture treatments, his back pain was erased. Throughout the following year, it would flare up on occasion, but would respond quickly to one or two more treatments. An occasional treatment from a chiropractor also proved helpful for him, and over time, he chose a routine of seeing me monthly for "tune-ups."

Then one day, after about a year and a half, he told me, for the first time, that for thirty years he had suffered from intense bowel urgency whenever he was nervous. On his way to social events like a party or to his part-time job, he would suddenly feel a desperate need to find the nearest restroom. As a safeguard, he and his wife had memorized the locations of all the public restrooms on their usual routes to vacation destinations and the homes of their friends. Rick had been reluctant to inform me about this before, but the problem had become severe enough that he had decided to finally tell me. Fortunately, two acupuncture treatments eliminated this bowel urgency and he was thrilled at this improvement. So Rick's back and his digestion were in fine shape after years of struggling with both.

One day, Rick came in for his monthly appointment to speak excitedly about a high school reunion he had just attended. He was incredulous, he said, hearing the torrent of medical complaints from his former high school classmates and seeing how much they had deteriorated. While he himself was happy and free of pain, everyone else was complaining about one serious medical problem or another. In contrast, he had become healthier and happier in the last two years and had gotten off his medications. Biologically, Rick had become a younger man in the last two years. He had been deflated at seventy-five, but now lively and energetic at seventy-seven. As he got a little older, he became a lot better.

The belief that we can become healthier isn't enough to change us, but it's an excellent first step. The hypothesis is worth testing. Countless seniors who previously blamed aging for their exhaustion and pain become happier and livelier as they age. They just needed to pull the correct levers of change.

The persistent ones

To imagine what's possible in our later years is to improve the chances of a better life. A telling reminder comes from the stories of centenarians, living emblems of the durability of healing potential.

In 2007, Canada, France, Japan, and the U.S. had a combined 175,000 citizens who were over a hundred years old. Such statistics can be overstated and often hard to verify, but even if the figure were off by 50 percent, we'd have a sizable subgroup of durable people. The Gerontology Research Group keeps a list of centenarians as well as super-centenarians, or people over a hundred and ten years old. The list notes that the person who lived the longest was Jeanne Calment, a French woman who lived a hundred and twenty-two years.

Then, in the book *The Blue Zones*, Dan Buettner describes research in four geographical areas with unusually high concentrations of centenarians: the Barbagio region of Sardinia, Italy; the Nicoya region of Costa Rica; the Seventh-day Adventist community of Loma Linda, California; and Okinawa, Japan. Each of these places has a disproportionately high number of centenarians who are not tenuously alive but lively. They eat whole foods, get plenty of sleep, and surround themselves with family and community. They hike, bike, garden, or lift weights, and otherwise keep physically active. They also laugh a lot.

Helen Klein of Rancho Cordova, California, started running after retiring at the age of fifty-five and got hooked. The first time she went out to run, all she could manage was two laps around a track of two-fifths of a mile. But before long, she was running five- and ten-kilometer races. Eventually, she became strong enough that throughout her sixties, seventies, and eighties, she broke age-group records for dozens of marathons and for ultramarathons, which are races of either fifty or a hundred miles. She completed the daunting Ironman

Triathlon, and at seventy-two, finished the 1995 Discovery Eco-Challenge in the desert Southwest, in which each team mountain-biked, rafted in white water, ran, and mountaineered for three hundred miles over five days. For the last event, she climbed a one-thousand foot sheer cliff in four hours. She'd never climbed in that manner before. It took most of her teammates only two hours to complete the climb, but they were in their twenties and thirties. At eighty-four, when I met her, she was running a marathon a month. Then, a year later, in 2008, she shattered the marathon world record of six hours and fifty-three minutes in her age group by over an hour—in a race where records are usually broken by a few minutes.

The well-known Jack LaLanne was a pistol who died at ninety-six. When he was seventy, after being handcuffed and shackled, he swam towing seventy people in seven boats for a mile and a half in Long Beach Harbor, California.

At ninety-one, Olga Kotelko held twenty-three world records in her age group for events like the high jump, long jump, javelin throw, shot put, and hundred-meter dash. Additionally, people in their eighties and nineties run in the marathons of New York, Boston, and other cities throughout the world.

To be healthy, we don't need to become supermen and superwomen running marathons and climbing cliffs in our eighties. With the enormous amounts of time and discipline required, the price of admission to this much stamina and strength is higher than most of us are willing or able to pay. It may be reassuring to hear that many studies indicate that much benefit can be had with modest exercise.

In fact, recent research has suggested that extremes in training might damage the heart. Those who run the most marathons and ultramarathons have had, according to some studies, a higher degree of cardiac fibrosis, or scarring, than the average athlete. But I mention Helen, Jack, and Olga because they're emblematic of the possibilities, because they splinter our assumptions about what's possible in old age. The extraordinary feats of these and other elders are reminders of the lions and tigers and bears of vitality sleeping in our flesh and bones. It's just that most of us haven't done what it takes to call those creatures out of their cozy beds. At virtually any stage of our lives, we would see remarkable changes in our health and moods if we were to devote one to two hours to age-appropriate exercise five to six days a week. I'm not suggesting that everyone do that much exercise, but those needing a serious makeover from miserable to merry, or those seeking high-level fitness, may need to do as much if they hope for a transformative change. Even when we've been exhausted and sickly for months or years, the seeds of possibility are still alive. Dormant, maybe, but alive.

The promise

One of the great advantages of tapping into the wellspring of healing is that it produces impeccable results with no side effects. When nature waves its wand, the outcomes are beautifully coordinated. No toll is exacted on other resources of the body. On the other hand, man-made substitutes for nature's wisdom always have side effects to one degree or another. As we've seen, under many circumstances, this is a worthy trade-off or the only solution, and often a life-saving necessity. But since the scientific perspective doesn't yet trust the primacy of our intrinsic healing power, we have come to rely too heavily on external sources of healing, on attempts to command nature (control and substitute). While this plays an invaluable role in medicine, an obsession with dominating nature can overshadow the high artistry of the body's intrinsic healing power. There we have an incomplete medicine—not wrong, but curtailed. We risk losing the skill of listening to nature's beating heart.

A corollary to all this is that we are responsible for our health. If we accept the job of coaxing out this healing potential, we'll need to work: to put in the extra time and effort to make a salad instead of grabbing a hot-dog; to go out for exercise though our bodies prefer to be a lump on the couch; to buy a gym membership instead of a new stereo; to have fruit instead of chocolate cake for dessert. Though we hear a lot about prevention today, the idea is now anemic—avoiding illness is smart but uninspired. What's more exciting is the vision of a medicine that awakens our potential to thrive, blossom, flourish, that helps us recognize that we are our own best healers and that we stand at the still center of the spinning, perplexing carousel of health.

I struggle to find words vivid enough to convey the beauty and magnitude of what's under our noses: this astonishing wellspring of healing, grace, and power that we find shimmering, breathing, and quivering in six and a half billion people, in countless plants, animals, trees, and grasses. As the ancient Taoists said, it's in the ten thousand things. This points not just to nature but to its fountainhead—the blueprint for the blueprint, the code for the code. We can see its signs in the blade of grass implausibly insinuating itself through a crack in a Manhattan sidewalk, in the lone cypress gripping nothing but rock on a coastal California cliff, in the bubbling spring water rising from the dark caverns of the earth, in the red and purple coral at the bottom of a turquoise sea, in the extravaganza of sex, birth, and death on the Serengeti plains, in a baby's crown emerging from the womb, and most of all, in the ceaseless human longing for the fleeting tastes of elation and redemption, for the next long exhalation, the absolute release, the next moment in which the promise of being human seems fulfilled and we no longer need to strive.

Name it what we will—the Tao, perennial wisdom, Mother Nature, the sacred universe, Brahman, the evolutionary impulse—it's trustworthy. It will be there to pick us up after school. To participate in its ways, first, we can remember the promise of creation lying in every cell of the body, every blink of the eye, every breath we take. Then we can act accordingly. Simple, but not easy. A good way to feel and know this promise is to look at the moon and stars and to think of what created all this. Whatever it was, it's not only outside and out there. It's in here too. It's waiting for us. Always.

Chapter Four

Health as Transformation, Medicine as Catalyst

At its core, health is one face of transformation. When Pablo Neruda wrote, "I want to do with you what spring does to the cherry tree," he gave us an image that captures the heart of this idea. Similarly, Nikos Kazantzakis wrote, "I said to the almond tree, 'Sister, speak to me of God,' and the almond tree blossomed." Health is not what remains after we correct a problem; it's more than the useful but now slightly feeble notion of prevention. It's not a static state. Instead, it's the flowering of human possibility that occurs in the way springtime draws out cherry and almond blossoms. The pink and white of the flowers are not solutions for a problem. When a small seed grows into a big chiseled tree, nothing was fixed. The seed was all blueprint, pure potential, only needing the right nourishment to sprout and reach for the clouds and to manifest its gift. So it is with a human being on the often-arduous passage from infant to elder, becoming someone who, in the end, bears virtually no resemblance to how she looked and behaved as a baby.

Health includes being joyful, energetic, conscious, and authentic. It's the harvest that follows tilling, planting, and reaping in the terrains of body and spirit. It depends on respecting those ingenious messages called symptoms, whether they're subtle as an itch or blatant as a migraine. As we've seen, health is not about band-aids and substitutions, but about evoking our power to become a force of wellness and inner beauty. The rational scientific mind is clearly necessary for the evolution of medicine and society, but the intuitive mind is better suited to savor, digest, and absorb the full meaning of a multidimensional vision of health and wellness. The image of the flowering almond or cherry tree conveys a world of meaning beyond the descriptive abilities of logic and reason. An integrative medicine includes both mind and heart, science and art, medicine and poetry, logos and eros.

The story of my patient Catherine will give you a glimpse into the idea that the search for health is often a journey toward wholeness.

Catherine was a bright, warm, and well-educated professional who had retired some years earlier. I'd guess that during her working years, her clients had enjoyed her comforting presence and easy laugh. But now, as the years rolled by, she was feeling progressively worse. On her health questionnaire, she wrote, "I can never remember a time when I have felt free of pain." Although the pain affected her entire body, it was most severe in one hip and one shoulder. During her first visit, I recommended that she start exercising, drink more than her usual two cups of water a day, drink less wine, reduce processed foods like desserts and snack foods, eat more vegetables, more fruit, and use the healthy oils such as olive oil and omega-3 found in salmon and other cold-water fish. While her sedentary life and dietary deficits were not the cause of her pains, they were most likely a major influence. Corrections in those areas would improve the chances of her feeling better.

Then, at one point during this first visit, after we had discussed her physical problems and her health history, Catherine began talking about the death of her adult daughter. Losing a child is the heartbreak to end all others, and Catherine's pain, still fresh after five years, was to be expected. She wept as she described her daughter's struggle with cancer and eventual death. Later, she said that while her grief would still sweep over her on occasion, the sense of loss no longer weighed on her life as it once had.

As we continued with acupuncture over the weeks, her energy increased, she lost weight, her hip felt better, and her shoulder pain went away. For the first time since she could remember, she would wake up without hurting all over. Her weight was melting off effortlessly. She was pleased with her progress. But then when she came for her sixth visit in as many weeks, she didn't mention her physical symptoms. Instead, she seemed agitated, speaking about her continual conflicts with her mother. It seemed that over the weeks, as her physical symptoms receded, her unfinished emotional work was moving to the top of the list. Then, during her next visit, she walked in, dropped into the chair, and grunted, "I don't feel peaceful." When I inquired into this, she started to cry and spoke of the distress she felt about this painful relationship with her mother. This in turn was related to her feeling overwhelmed from caring for everyone's needs but her own, which also kept her from spending time with her husband. As the process of healing peeled away more layers of the onion, her grief over her daughter's death, and her weariness from hiding that pain from the world, emerged in full.

As our pains decrease or disappear, and as we become more alive, the evolutionary push from within will thrust forward with more aplomb. If a patient finds her pains and other symptoms improving, only to face the emergence of emotional distress, she's usually progressing. It feels bad, but is good. It's catharsis at work, or abreaction, to be more precise. Usually, it's a surprise to the patient—how can the evaporation of physical pains lead to emotional distress? Fortunately, Catherine was intuitive enough to understand that these feelings were unfinished business. "They've been there," she said knowingly. She knew that her daughter's death was a profound, unspeakable loss that had left its signature on her psyche. She recognized the need to stop caring for others at the expense of her vitality and peace. In the past, she had worked on these concerns in psychotherapy, being fully aware of their effect on her life. But years later, as soon as her physical pains decreased through acupuncture, the sadness came out of the wings and took center stage. It wasn't finished with her yet. As we discussed how the emergence of these painful emotions was a good step forward, she agreed. She knew that the discomfort was prodding her to grow.

When the body heals from the ground up, unfinished business often emerges. As pain exits the body, unresolved grief, fear, or anger can take their rightful place. The reason for this is that emotional pain often seeks refuge in the body's weak links. In my observations over the years, it seems that what's most likely to emerge is sadness or grief, with anger a close second. Tenacious, waiting for years or even decades, the unfinished business waits in the caverns of the unconscious. It will not capitulate in its need to be on full display, to be known, heard, and then put to rest. When denied a full hearing, an unresolved emotion becomes opportunistic, looking for vulnerable spots like a disc herniation here, a cardiac insufficiency there, a dormant virus here. It will then raise a ruckus, with the strategy of grabbing our attention. If we won't resolve the grief, fear, or anger through direct, conscious work, then it will recruit any body part as its spokesperson. If, on the other hand, we can muster the courage to work through the regurgitation and the muck of deep emotional work, the body is left alone to be light and clear. Until then, the loose dangling ends will wave frantically to get our attention. The back, neck, knees, shoulders, bowels, lungs, liver, pancreas, stomach, adrenals—they're all vulnerable; they're all fair game. If they don't get the closure they want, they might explode. Here is Harlem [2] from Langston Hughes:

What happens to a dream deferred?

> Does it dry up
> Like a raisin in the sun?
> Or does it fester like a sore —
> And then run?

Does it stink like rotten meat?
Or crust and sugar over —
Like a syrupy sweet?
Maybe it just sags
Like a heavy load.

Or does it explode?

The purpose of symptoms is to help us heal, grow, transform into an integrated, whole, vibrant human being. They originate in the wisdom and the powers that created the earth, in the *anima mundi*—the soul of the world. Once they have lost their oblique avenues of self-expression—the physical outlets for emotional pain—they come into the sunlight of direct awareness. At those moments, we can choose to face our grief, humiliation, loneliness, or rage—a task requiring immense courage—or we can ignore them and have them sink again into the dark muted corners of the unconscious. Of course, many symptoms are only physical. But many are amplifiers for the voice of prisoners in the subconscious self.

Unfortunately, we too often misinterpret the traffic on the bidirectional highway between mind and body as a problem in need of a remedy. Whether through medications, herbs, denial, overwork, alcohol, or other methods, we scramble to blunt the symptom without first trying to understand its purpose. But though the symptom masquerades as a problem, it's really a hint. It's precisely our pain and our grief that lead us forward on the trail of healing.

Our mandate in these moments is to unload the burden of unwept tears, of emulsified anger, of unspeakable pain and fear, of any unfinished emotional work. In many situations, the well-intentioned dispensing of anti-depressants or sedatives only delays the collision with emotions that eventually leads to healing and integration. While psychological integration often requires more than just catharsis and abreaction, becoming fully aware of fugitive emotions is a great start. Catherine was being nudged forward to heal her relationship with her mother and to work further on her grief. She was given little choice once her physical pains began to dissolve.

Another story will illustrate a similar pattern of healing. Linda was a fifty-eight-year-old account executive with piercing, unremitting pain in her right groin, hip, and lower back. Despite cortisone injections and pain medications from her doctors, the ferocious pain had refused to budge. After we discussed the nature and the history of her pain, I asked if she was under stress. She answered that since she hated her job, she suspected her work-related stresses of exaggerating her pain. With the combination of distress about her work and her physical pains, she was being shoved against the walls of her endurance.

After we discussed her health history, her lifestyle, and other circumstances of her life, I had her lie on the treatment table. I then inserted a few acupuncture needles, which she hardly felt, and left her for the usual thirty minutes. When I returned, she was crying. She said that while I'd been out of the room, her pain had reduced by half. But as it decreased, she also saw that the real source of her stress wasn't her job. Instead, it was the longing to be with all her children and grandchildren who lived thousands of miles away.

As we continued with treatments weekly over the next two months, her pains steadily subsided while her spirits continued to rise. We were both pleased with her progress. Then, in the eighth week, she walked into the treatment room, flopped into the chair, glared at me, and said, "David, what are you doing to me? I've been crying all week since the last treatment." I told her that she might be in the next phase of healing, that hidden emotions might be surfacing. I took her pulses—the twelve we read in acupuncture—and the qualities were excellent. From being low, weak, and debilitated at her first visit, they had become robust, alive, and balanced. (On the radial arteries on both wrists, we read qualities in twelve different pulses. They're categorized into twenty-eight different conditions such as soggy, wiry, choppy, slippery, floating, sinking, etc.) The energy of the earth was flowing strongly in her body; her pulses were in outstanding shape.

I then asked how her pain was, and she replied, "It's completely gone." Eight weeks ago, it had been an ogre, and now it was nowhere in sight. So I repeated the idea that when pains go away, unfinished emotions can resurface. Did she think this might be happening to her? After an awkward pause, she said, "I wasn't going to tell you this. But memories of being sexually abused at eight years old have been coming to me all week."

She had spent years in psychotherapy and a little time in hypnotherapy working on this, so she had thought it was all behind her. Consciously, it hadn't been a problem for her in years. But when her physical pains vanished, the long fingers of painful memories reached out after fifty years, hopefully for their last grasp. Over the following month, she worked through the remnants of these memories easily, and in short order, felt terrific. Within a few months, she quit her job and moved with her husband to live near her grandchildren.

The stories of Catherine and Linda tell us that their pains came *through*, not *from*, their nerves, muscles, and joints. On the other hand, were the pains only psychological, only psychosomatic? Unlikely. The impulse of unresolved emotions takes advantage of perforations in the armor of our anatomy and physiology, seeking the spots that then become physical speaker systems for blaring the message.

Though the unfinished business took advantage of Linda's and Catherine's weak links, it was not the cause of the pain, as usually envisioned in the notion of a single cause leading to a single effect. The pain needed a vulnerable physiological spot. As we saw in the story of the broken window, the idea of a single cause is less than useful when we look at the complexity of the whole and its many streams of influence. Emotions dissolve into the physical self like salt into water.

What was being asked of Linda and Catherine was metamorphosis, a transmutation of straw into gold. As the evolutionary impulse moved through their symptoms, it coerced them to find their truth, to heal. If the symptoms could speak, they might have said: flower, grow, blossom.

In his *Sonnets to Orpheus*, Rilke told us to whisper, in the presence of immeasurable darkness, *I'm flowing* to the silent earth, and to say I am to the flashing water. This affirms the spirit of deep healing, even when faced with the bitterest loss imaginable. Our symptoms help us get there.

There are a thousand ways in which we are challenged to evolve. They are necessary confrontations with what makes us stronger, more resilient, more authentically ourselves. Conversely, avoiding these encounters can lead to the paradoxical result of worsening our health. A strategy to vanquish pain without understanding its meaning is incomplete and possibly harmful.

The evolutionary push behind our symptoms demands that we be more awake. It needs us to know the depths of our souls, to live fully, to live authentically. True vitality requires us to be genuine, to feel our emotions entirely, which may, from time to time, require a crisp new courage as we drop into the dark cellars of our pain. If we assume this task, then we'll have taken a big step toward wholeness.

As we continue to explore new ways of understanding medicine and health, here's a quick look at how we normally think of them.

The remedial view of medicine

The view both on the street and in academia is that medicine's purpose is to fix problems. One underlying principle is that you're either healthy or you're not, as measured by standard tests. So the sequence goes like this: we're fine and healthy until we get sick, then we get fixed, and then we're back to the norm of being healthy. Being healthy is defined as a condition without disease. This diagram illustrates the model:

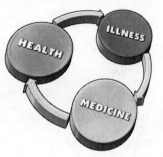

In this view, the role of medicine is purely remedial. Its purpose is to repair what's broken and restore the patient to her previous condition. In emergency conditions where quick, potent interventions are required, this of course is essential. As we saw in the last chapter, the methods of a remedial model are invaluable for their intended purposes. But for wellness, for vitality, we need a more nuanced model.

If we watch and listen closely, we'll see that our bodies constantly move through the many shades of gray between wellness and illness. We're never in a static condition, but always a little more energetic one day, a little less the next, a little achy one day, a little better the next. It's helpful to pay attention to these subtle changes, as they are feedback on how well we're taking care of our physical and emotional health. As subjective measures, they're usually accurate indications of what's going on in our energy systems and our blood chemistry.

In my attempt to further describe these ideas, I'll first sidestep briefly to give a little background on a philosophical idea. It may help in learning to perceive the body not as a solid object like a rock, but as a form of energy in constant change, like a river.

Rivers of change

The ancient Greek philosopher Heraclitus is known for saying you can never step into the same river twice. All things are in constant flux, he said, and since the water in the river changes constantly, we step into a different river each time. As another way of illustrating this idea, he said that everything was made of fire, the primordial element of the world. He wrote, "This world... was ever, is now, and ever shall be, eternal fire." What he meant is simply that all things are endlessly changing.

Several thousand miles east in India, the Buddha taught that impermanence, anicca, is a characteristic of all that exists, whether it's a thought or a mood, a rock or a butterfly. Well over two thousand years before the discovery of the electron microscope, he stated that all matter was made of atoms—and that one of their characteristics was constant motion. The Greek philosophers Leucipus and Democritus also theorized that atoms were the smallest bits of matter. In India long before the heyday of the Greek philosophers, Ayurvedic medicine thought of the human body as an aggregate of energy, not as a collection of physical parts.

Further east yet, Lao Tzu and the theorists of Chinese medicine spoke of the forces of life as a pulsing energy, constantly moving and cycling endlessly between *yin* and *yang*. The body was energy, they said, not a thing. This life force, the *qi*, reflected the moods of nature as they shifted from summer to winter, hot to cold, loud to quiet, light to darkness. This idea of constant change between polar opposites is expressed equally in the dance between intimacy and coldness, love and indifference, joy and sorrow. But the common thread here is that the human body was seen not as a collection of organs, but of processes. It wasn't a thing, but a cascade of energy that happens to look and feel solid.

In more contemporary times, physicists have been insisting since the early 1900s that matter is not made of matter. Instead, it's a collection of energy patterns in the form of subatomic particles whirling and banging about. In the twenty-first century, when quantum physicists describe subatomic particles as possibilities rather than things, they're not allegorizing or being disingenuous.

From the perspective of quantum physics, a rigorously mathematical discipline, the body is not a block of insentient matter—just as the ancient wisdom traditions tell us. Instead, it's a possibility. To repeat, the body is a possibility, not a thing. Einstein's famous formula, $E=mc2$, means that energy is equal to matter times the square of the speed of light. This means that matter equals energy, and this energy is always in motion—a statement that's not simile or analogy, but pure literal science.

I suspect it will seem strange, or at least curious, to think of our flesh and bones as processes instead of things, as verbs instead of nouns, as possibilities instead of objects. Our senses tell us otherwise when we bump our heads on the cupboard. But the body is perpetually changing, not only from year to year or day to day, but from one billionth of a second to the next.

On the biological scale, our red blood cells are completely replaced every hundred and twenty days. We have a new liver every seven years. In quantum physics, it's known that subatomic particles, including those of our bodies, dissolve and vanish billions of times every second, followed by the birth of new ones that look just like the old ones. Where they go to and come from, no one knows. Physicists refer to it as the quantum void. But most relevant for our purposes is the felt experience of change, the nonstop Ferris wheel of sensations in our minds and bodies.

On some days, we're energetic and on top of our game. On others, we're tired and can't do anything right. One morning, you might wake up achy and lethargic. Maybe a little better after that breakfast diet soda or high-test coffee. Sleepy after lunch while facing down a boring spreadsheet. Then anxious about a looming deadline. Uplifted by a good word from the boss. Tired in the evening at home, maybe a little moody. Then your two-year-old says "I love you, Mommy" for the first time, and you are elated beyond words. Feelings and sensations change like the passing landscape during a train ride through the Rockies.

With a careful look at this emotional and physical terrain, we'll find hundreds of shades in subjective human experience. Every physical or emotional feeling has a unique fingerprint, each dissimilar to the previous one, just as we'd find every water molecule in the river of Heraclitus different from the others. It might be less joyful and more poignant. Or the back pain might ache more but burn less.

Those individuals who are struggling with pain, fatigue, or any other symptom would notice, with close attention, that the sensations change day to day, hour to hour, and often minute to minute. And then, regardless of their nature, they can change dramatically in a flash. Between awful and sublime, the shades of gray are many.

In the big picture, then, remembering the constancy of change helps in breaking up the static idea that we're either healthy or we're not. It helps us see health as a humming, breathing, pulsing condition changing from one moment to the next—amorphous, fluid, twisting, winding—just like clouds on a windy day or the moods of a toddler.

Let's take one step further now and look even more closely at the nature of these changes.

Shades of gray

So if health and disease sit on a continuum with many shades of gray, what do these shades look like? The following chart illustrates a set of broad categories.

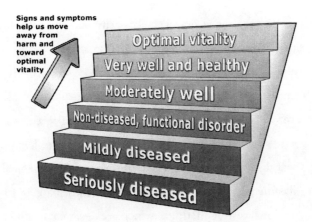

Spectrum of conditions between health and disease

Tucked between these categories, we'll find many more nuanced shades of health. It's a far cry from the idea that we're either sick or we're not.

One idea related to this can reassure many people suffering from conditions that defy diagnosis. It's called a functional disorder, a condition for which a medical diagnosis can't be found but is nevertheless uncomfortable or painful. No matter if people feel terrible or only slightly sick, medical tests such as blood tests, MRIs, CAT scans, and other studies show no signs of anything gone awry. But the suffering is still present. These problems are sometimes considered psychosomatic, but while the psychological face of symptoms is always involved to one degree or another, the common saying that it's all in your head is an outdated one.

A simple way to understand a functional disorder is through this analogy: think of how you can feel exhausted, stressed, and just plain awful at the end of a bad day at work or a frenzied day taking care of the kids. It doesn't mean you're sick. You happen to feel bad, but you're not diseased.

Similarly, your liver can be tired and stressed, so to speak, after a pounding from excessive alcohol, sugar, and unhealthy fats. When only occasionally pushed too far, it doesn't necessarily become pathologically ill. Now, it certainly can become pathological if this pattern continues. But you as a whole, like your individual internal organs, can be stressed without being sick. So in a similar though more noticeable way, your body can feel ill, and sometimes severely so, with a functional disorder even in the absence of a pathology. You're simply operating below optimum levels of health.

A functional disorder is real even without supporting medical evidence of disease or dysfunction. The roots of the feelings just happen to be out of range of conventional testing methods, which are designed to find pathology, not these subtle shadings in our subjective experience. Even if all those aches and pains and other symptoms were "psychosomatic," they are still and always a message that something, somewhere, needs to be corrected. In light of what we discussed in Chapter Two, a functional disorder is simply a set of symptoms trying to help us to change course.

Many CAM therapies such as homeopathy, acupuncture, osteopathic manipulation, chiropractic, herbal medicine, massage, naturopathy, bodywork, and nutrition counseling are often able to find the reasons behind these functional disorders. They use diagnostic maps broad enough to identify and correct subtle, non-pathological imbalances.

Some medical doctors practice what's now called functional medicine, an approach using diet, nutritional supplements, and other natural therapies to help finely tune a patient's blood chemistry. This in essence has long been the domain of the naturopath, but is now becoming more popular with a small percentage of physicians.

Short of an identifiable pathology, many functional disorders are the result of minor deficiencies or excesses in blood chemistry. If lab readings of estrogen, thyroid hormone, potassium, or blood sugar are only leaning slightly toward abnormal, your sense of wellbeing can suffer. Correction is possible through the dietary changes and nutritional supplements recommended by the doctors and other practitioners using functional medicine. Since one idea in integrative medicine is that no one is in perfect balance, these subtle imbalances are worth identifying and correcting. As trends or patterns, they might be forecasting disease in the distant future.

So now with some background in the fluidity of the human experience, the porous borders between health and illness, and the marriage of mind and body, we can begin to further explore the idea of health as transformation.

Growl, grit, and growth

Poets, playwrights, novelists, artists, and composers—from Aeschylus to Albee, Liszt to Lennon, Raphael to Rothko—have spoken over the millennia of the human drama with its many faces of triumph and tragedy. Whether through music, dance, the visual arts, or the written word, these stories sensitize us to the perils of the human predicament and then to the requisites for their transcendence. They captivate us as they reach into the most evocative places of the soul.

Then we have the slavish attention paid to movie stars, singers, and rock stars. These icons of human possibility, even if they live up to our ideals only on screen or on stage, are irresistible to many. But this magnetic pull is more than just prurience, projection, lust, or envy. Both drama and those who portray it well are alluring for their truth-telling, their boldness in portraying both the darker side of the soul and the luminous face of the heroic self. But this is truth-telling not as in a scientific true or false, but as in the human soul laid bare—whether what emerges is noble or disgraceful. When we watch and identify with the movie hero who eventually transcends cowardice, ambivalence, or narcissism, we are brought closer to our own authentic core— the audacious, heroic, transformational self. We are then made more real and more alive.

Granted, drama can be mere indulgence. But the enduring stories of heroism, revealing the human heart at its best, jolt us awake with their gritty texture. They stir the longings for own unbridled aliveness. With the drift in our culture toward living in the clouds of artifice, we aren't often encouraged to plumb the depths of our souls. But getting there can turn the soul Technicolor, which then helps us become healthier.

If a story has the protagonist cakewalk to his glorious ending, we'd be bored—it wouldn't be a story. Instead, we're riveted when our hero encounters something growling on the road ahead, leaving us in suspense about his willingness and his ability to vanquish the monster—contemporary or mythic, organic or corporate. In line with a mythological view of human dilemmas, conquest here is metaphor for the transformation of the self from fearful to brave, selfish to selfless.

The great mythologist Joseph Campbell wrote beautifully about myths as lessons for inner transformation. He wrote that myths, from all cultures and times, represent universal truths about the nature of the cosmos and the human experience. They illustrate the necessity of love, courage, selflessness, loyalty, and the like if we are to live fully and wholly. He said that myths, far from being mere flights of fancy, are teaching tools for the spiritual journey. In particular, he noted that all cultures have myths describing the hero's journey, the sacred quest—a motif he found surprisingly similar throughout the world.

In these stories, the hero is first drawn by the irresistible appeal of a beautiful princess, a treasure, or some other wonder. After he learns of this great possibility, which represents his soul's fulfillment, he leaves the comfort of the castle to start his journey. Inevitably, he encounters a life-threatening challenge in the form of a malevolent being. But then, by calling upon his reserves of strength, cunning, and courage, he kills or tricks this diabolical opponent. At this point, he is free to find the princess, treasure, or other reward—which represents his spiritual actualization.

Campbell said that the people and other creatures in mythology represent parts of ourselves. The hero's encounter with things that hiss, growl, snap, or snarl reflects the confrontation with the shadow elements within ourselves. Killing the monster or other antagonist represents the transcendence of these limitations as well as others such as cynicism, resignation, fear of risk, fear of failing, fear of embarrassment. On the hero's journey, we have little choice but to destroy the monster if we are to be granted the objects of our desire that represent transcendence and spiritual wholeness. This transformation can only take place by having the courage to first face and then overcome our challenges.

What's the relevance of all this to medicine and health? It's a literary take on the idea that the symptom is a message encouraging us to grow. The purpose of the journey is health and fulfillment, and the symptoms are both the call to start on this journey and the obstacles to be overcome. By engaging in the challenges along the way, we are transformed. In the end, our health and optimal vitality are inseparable from the path of transformation, as it includes the psychological, social, and spiritual elements of the human experience.

The waltz between the light and the shadow is the matrix of growth. It's precisely this vacillation that becomes the stuff of transformation. While literature is replete with this theme, and while we teach it to our children, we haven't fully embodied it as individuals or as a culture. We still act as if the obstacles are nuisances to be ignored.

For a long time it had seemed to me that life was about to begin—real life. But there was always some obstacle in the way, something to be gotten through first, some unfinished business, time still to be served, a debt to be paid. Then life would begin. At last it dawned on me that these obstacles were my life.

–Alfred D. Souza

Cheryl came to me with severe, debilitating pain in her lower back. When she first came, her walk was slow and hesitant. As she slowly lowered herself into the chair, her misery was evident. On the health questionnaire, she had rated her pain a ten out of ten, the worst you can imagine, so I suggested she get onto the treatment table if that would be more comfortable. As she carefully worked herself onto it, she grimaced often but eventually managed to lie on her back. As we continued to talk, I told her that in some cases, unfinished emotional concerns can surface as pain decreases. Cheryl acknowledged that such emotions might in fact emerge for her. But her most urgent concern was getting rid of her back pain.

After the treatment, her pain was greatly reduced. When she returned the next week, the improvement had lasted; after the second treatment, the pain was reduced even further. But when she came for her third visit, she said she'd been crying all week since the treatment, which incidentally had eliminated most of the pain.

Once the pain was gone, all the unresolved torment of her life had come flooding into her conscious awareness. She had cried for hours during the week, overcome by a tidal wave of the emotional turmoil of her past: her father's coldness and cruelty, perhaps related to the major loss of life during World War II that occurred under his command; her mother's addiction to appearances and propriety; her two divorces; the years of her charade as the perfect corporate wife; the ache of an existential loneliness; crushing doubts about her self-worth; and her sense of being abandoned by God. As it all rushed forth, she cried a rain shower.

After she spoke for a while, I suggested once again that this storm of emotions might be the next step in her healing, that while she felt awful, she was improving. Without the distracting noise of back pain, her emotions were now thrust before the glaring stage lights, insisting on resolution. She agreed. She'd spent her entire life avoiding these issues, she said, by keeping herself distracted and staying constantly busy and overworked. But she still didn't want to face them because they were too painful and overwhelming. Though she knew she had traded her back pain for this, she wanted to run. Through her tears, she looked at me and said, "Can I have my pain back?" We both burst out laughing.

At a speech in Indianapolis announcing the assassination of Martin Luther King, Jr. on April 4, 1968, Robert F. Kennedy quoted this from Aeschylus:

In our sleep,

pain which cannot forget

falls drop by drop upon the heart

until, in our own despair,

against our will, comes wisdom

through the awful grace of God.

Aeschylus wrote of the wisdom waiting behind our unassailable grief, and by proxy, behind all our pains. Healing on the spiritual journey often comes from pain that surgically incises the soul for access to what helps us heal and evolve. The pain rips wide open the skin of the soul, but for the benevolent purpose of helping us heal and integrate. Cheryl's feelings, against her will, were now fully revealed. They were pushing her headlong into the healing and wisdom coming from an awful grace.

Hardwired

While no one would admit to the naïve notion that life should be a cruise, we're neurologically hardwired to want it so. In addition, we've been culturally trained to dismiss pain quickly without thinking about its backhanded, slanted messages. No one taught us to consider our pain the very force that drives us forward in our development and transformation—whether physical, psychological, or spiritual. Through the unconscious propaganda of both instinct and culture, we've been trained to hope the pain will summarily disappear.

A good portion of the psyche's drive is aimed at survival and pleasure. It corresponds mostly to the animalistic part of the brain called the limbic system, sometimes known as the reptilian brain. With little regard for civility or justice, it's focused on only the basics of survival, procreation, and relevant actions like eating, running, and killing. Today, we redirect this primitive drive into financial, social, political, and psychological survival. We go acrobatic trying to fulfill these needs, and at our worst, we deny, deceive, manipulate, dominate, steal, and even take life to survive.

Though our rational selves can accept the inevitability of suffering, we scurry when pain knocks on the door, driven by primal, animal instinct. We live, breathe, and sleep our desire for stability and security. We have the impossible and subconscious wish for immunity from all we consider undesirable, not that we'd readily admit to it. But if we would stop waging war against symptoms and become curious about their logic and their message, we'd rise above instinct and ultimately improve the odds of becoming well. To clarify this idea a little more, here's a parallel.

Muscles, energy, and growth of the psyche

Before a muscle can become stronger, it must be stressed. It must be pushed to a point of exertion where the muscle fibers are destroyed. You know you're there when you feel the burn during your workout. At that point, you're consuming the energy stored in the muscles, roughly similar to the way fire consumes a log. When energy in a log is released through fire, the result is actualized energy in the form of heat. But with our muscles, the energy is translated into actions like cycling, dancing, running, building a house, or repairing a car.

Fortunately, the body responds to this good stress as designed: it automatically builds new muscle once it gets rest and healthy food. This is the natural, automatic consequence to the destruction of muscle fibers. In the big picture, destruction is part of the cycle leading to greater physical strength.

The same is true of aerobic capacity. When we push ourselves beyond the comfort zone in our cardio workouts, we increase endurance. In these scenarios, the swing between yin and yang is the theater of growth and better health. It's the metabolic equivalent of the hero's journey.

We can also see this happening in the way the body metabolizes food. The process that creates energy bonds and new tissue from food is called anabolism, where molecules bind with each other to create larger molecules. In short, it's like building a new house. It puts pieces of a chemical puzzle together to create and build something new, and is essentially how we build bigger muscles and reserves of energy in the cells.

But before anabolism can occur, we need catabolism, which is the breaking down of tissues and energy bonds. It's what happens when a log is on fire, which is the release of energy formerly sequestered in the wood as the energy of heat and smoke. Rest, sleep, fats, and proteins support anabolism, while stress, insufficient food, too much sugar or carbohydrates, and exercise are catabolic. The extreme of the anabolic state is the bulging muscularity of professional bodybuilders, while the extreme catabolic state is found in the skin and bones of a spindly malnourished child in Somalia. To be healthy, we need a balance between anabolic and catabolic actions in the body. So again, we find another parallel in the human body to the way we grow psychologically and spiritually.

Health as transformation

From all this, we can see that health is far more than the absence of disease, but a transformative journey. It's the process of growing, becoming, developing.

It's about becoming the possible human.

If we are attentive, we can always feel in our bodies the yen for change, the longings that are just the impulse of the Kosmos pressing against the edges of our growth. In these sensations of the body, we find our betrothal to the world's wisdom. This impulse for change is also at work when spring calls forth the purple of the iris, the light green of a leaf, or the reds of an azalea. If our attention is strong and clear, we may be led to those rare moments when the doors of perception are thrown open and we become privileged and humbled to witness the iridescence of being dissolved into all that surrounds us, feeling for at least a few moments the evaporation of our identity as separate, isolated souls encapsulated on the inside of our skin.

Philosophers and spiritual teachers such as Teilhard de Chardin and Sri Aurobindo have written that an evolutionary impulse is embodied in the universe. In this model of evolution, which resembles Darwin's ideas only remotely, the universe is an integration of matter and consciousness. It's evolving toward greater wholeness and a conscious revelation, an end that de Chardin called the Omega point. Unlike Darwin's theory of evolution, which focuses only on biological change, this refers to a conscious and meaningful universe driven by an impulse found in both matter and consciousness.

What's most relevant for our health is that this conscious evolutionary impulse, this immeasurable grandness, speaks directly to us through our pain, pleasure, and our symptoms. It isn't a concept, but a living, pulsing vitality at work every second in every thought of the mind and every cell of the body. Whether we're feeling the warmth of love or the toxicity of resentment, we're having more than a "me" experience: we are feeling the full weight of this vast potentiality, this vitality, the drive to become, that has always existed everywhere. This means that even the most banal symptom like a stiff back or a headache is a direct communication from the miraculous intelligence that informs all of life itself. So how inelegant is it to ignore a personal message direct from the source of all life? Remembering the distinguished pedigree of a message like a stomachache or anxiety can help us treat it with respect and be more receptive to its instructions.

This view of health as transformation can lead to respect for the pain, the sorrow, and the hellish moments of human experience. Health is not about waging war against them, but embracing them. Whether in mythology or metabolism, the shadows must be included. The ups and downs of living are an integral part of the trajectory of growth. We knew that. But it's time to really know that. Beyond the pursuit of feeling good, we can think of medicine's ultimate purpose as assistance in helping us transform into the best we can be.

Learning from my symptoms

With regard to my own health, I wrote earlier that my symptoms were telling me to stay active. In looking at its deeper implications, I've since wondered if the pressure might be the analog of a repressed childhood. The pressure increased with stillness and decreased with movement. Was there a symbolic meaning in that?

If I felt trapped when the pressure was tight, was this redolent of being crammed into a mold by Catholic rules and the disciplines of my father? Maybe it was an archetypal pattern I'd inherited, maybe a random act of fate. Or, as my teachers at Kanduboda put it, it might have been the effect of karma, the brunt of the past on the present—which a solid morality and meditative practice should help. But it did occur to me that the pressure might be a relic of the viselike oppression I felt in my childhood.

As a child, I was sent to a Catholic school in Tokyo called St. Mary's International run by the Brothers of Christian Instruction of Canada, a happy coincidence for my father who was French Canadian by birth. Going to a Catholic school helped cast long shadows of guilt in my young mind. I grew up ashamed of everything—my body, my urges, my sin of anger toward my father—and felt flawed at the core.

Venial sins were milk bottles with a few stains, while mortal sins were milk bottles stained almost black. Accumulating enough of those darker bottles would earn me a spot in hell. Hell meant having flames scorching your skin for eternity, the worst part being you couldn't die from it. On earth, you'd die in minutes when engulfed in flames; down in the moral cellars of the universe, you'd be seared and roasted without end. I worried about that a lot. Burning my finger while lighting a firecracker or playing with matches was painful enough. Extrapolating that to hideous flames burning my entire body not for a few seconds, but forever, was the most horrific of thoughts. I couldn't imagine the pain of someone holding a match to my finger for one minute. But trillions of years with my entire body engulfed in fire? Are you kidding?

So for the most part, I was obedient and pious at school. I wasn't exactly a teacher's pet, but I got myself favored, assuming this might be a sort of insurance against the worst actuarial risk of my life. To further improve my odds, I'd often go to the chapel in the administration building and pray to the Virgin Mary before the school bus left for its hour-long trip back home to Grant Heights.

Mom was a shy beauty and the sweetest of women, but subservient. She was an unequal counterbalance for the militarism my father brought to marriage and parenthood. Unfortunately, his drill sergeant ways would kick in with the smallest infraction—what worked in running brigades and air raids and winning the whole world war ought to work at home too. It made fragile all periods of peace in the household.

On the good side, he was a fun-loving prankster prone to corny humor. And he was reliable: always at home, taking me to the beach, to the mountains to ski and hike. He didn't drink, smoke, gamble, or fritter away his money. His struggles through the Depression had cemented the already frugal habits learned during his early years on the poor streets of Sherbrooke, Quebec. This may have explained why he would sniff at the lack of any practical uses for art.

When crossed, Dad got rough. He often spanked me, hard, and yelled at me even more often. One of my frequent punishments was to kneel in the corner on the hardwood floor for a half-hour. Praying was optional. I just needed to feel my knees ache.

Decades after his death, a few of his twelve brothers and sisters told me that they had suggested he go easy on me and my two younger brothers, but to no effect. I was relieved to hear that I hadn't exaggerated his severity. Even during my years as a child, I could see how harshness and discipline were different. I knew it was the darts in his eyes and the knife-edges in his voice, and not the rules, that stung. I believe his words left a bigger bruise on my soul than his palms did on my stinging buttocks. Mom did her best to buffer and mediate, and when too late, to be the emotional nurse. Sometimes she got through to Dad, sometimes she didn't.

The harsh disciplinary life at home was, coincidentally, well coordinated with the induction of guilt and shame through my early catechism classes. Church dogma reduced to child-level comprehension was a setup for the repression of the natural impulses running about like a wild pony in a young boy's body and mind. Combined with the rules and discipline at home, a child could get caught in a double bind. There was no way out. In retrospect, I see the absence of an escape route as one of the more punishing elements of that time in my life.

One day, when I was about eight or nine, my father yelled at me and spanked me for some reason I've long forgotten. When I started crying and walking up the stairs to my bedroom, he came up from behind and spanked me hard again, shouting, "Stop crying! Stop crying!" I didn't know what to do with the illogic of the command. I remember feeling the anguish of the injustice, after which I said to myself, "I hate him. I hate him." As soon as the thought came, my anguish turned to horror: I'd just committed a mortal sin. My milk bottle was all black. It was bad enough feeling like a worm and having a father acting as if he hated me. But this new sin meant that if I died in an accident before I could rush to my next confession, I'd burn in hell forever. Which is more than a trillion years.

With the few options available to a child at times like this, he can choke it all down in the way a boa swallows a mouse. But it can turn into a lump in the psychological bowels where life is digested, becoming a drag on the healthy metabolism of emotions. Guilt and shame zipped my mouth shut, muzzling self-expression.

Years later, long after my hair had gone gray, I was sitting at the kitchen table when a corrective picture came to me. I saw myself as a small boy, crying, and screaming at him, "You have no right to touch this body without my permission."

Only a few months ago, I learned something else that may have fed the low self-esteem I felt in my earlier years. Shame within a family can, if you will, be absorbed through the air. While rummaging through my parents' old documents one day, I found their marriage certificate. It was dated four years after I was born. That explained why they never celebrated their wedding anniversary. It may be related to an extraordinary experience I had some fifteen years ago in a workshop. During a breathwork-induced altered state, I felt as though a lament of unbearable shame was being transferred from my mother to me during my birth.

My father was born in 1914, long before self-help books crammed bookstore shelves. He didn't stand a chance of dispelling his inner gremlins when the tools for such work hadn't been invented yet. As I got older, he and I came to understand each other better, but we would have grueling years ahead of us when I got to high school.

Toward the end of his life, our relationship healed, as I'll show in the last chapter. But at the time, especially with an eighth grade education, the best he could do was to follow the guidelines in the unwritten manuals he'd inherited from his parents, the Vatican, and the United States Army. Only decades later would parenthood benefit from the research on self-understanding, relationships, and child rearing. Whether it was the mechanical impact of his life on mine like one billiard ball clacking against another, or an archetypal transmission of his pent-up boiler-room energy, or both, it seemed likely that the pressure I felt as a child might have been reincarnated as the pressure on my head during my adult years.

During my time at St. Mary's, I also made a choice that presaged my decision to become a monk in Sri Lanka in later years. In the fifth grade, when Brother Peter lectured to us about the preeminence of being a brother like himself, his presentation was so compelling that I decided to go that route for my career. I was ten. At the least, being a brother sounded better than being a priest who had to memorize all that Latin. I was earnest about it, although the ambition would go up in a puff of smoke when I discovered girls and rock and roll a few years later. During those teen years, I became irate with the Church's dogma and tactics, but I've since come to appreciate Christianity in the more liberal theologies of writers like Thomas Merton, Pierre Teilhard de Chardin, and Matthew Fox.

In the late seventies and early eighties, after getting sick in Sri Lanka, restoring my health became the priority. The pressure then became a guiding force, directing me toward what was best for me. I found that when it released its grip a little, I'd start to feel angry toward my father. In retrospect, I see that the pressure was made, in part, of choked impulses and strangled self-expression.

In prior years, while I was still in undergraduate school, my need to break free of the chains of my childhood coincided with the waves of social turbulence in the sixties and early seventies. Before I started wearing monk robes, my clothing was that of a wild-haired hippie—garb for the nonconformist, for the rebel, for the freedom-seeker swayed by the cool of Jack Kerouac, the howling of Allen Ginsberg, the soothing tones of Ram Dass, and others rejecting what we saw as a skewed value system disfiguring the face of American society.

We found a sense of power in our angry rebuke of materialism, racism, stiff collars, xenophobia, the subjugation of women, sexual repression, ecological hubris, the aggressions of the White House and the Pentagon, and the straightjacket of Father-Knows-Best traditionalism in suburban America. We were outraged at the country's willingness to destroy millions of Vietnamese lives and to eventually lose fifty-five thousand of our own teenagers and men for dubious moral justifications and suspect geopolitical ends. The Domino Theory sounded hollow to us. It all left our generation frustrated with the prevailing political system and the country's values. We were boiling. During the summers between academic years, my friend George and I worked as construction laborers. One day, when the boss told us to demolish a wall of concrete block with sledge hammers, we tore it down with Viking zest, enjoying the chaos and feeling exhilarated from releasing our pent-up energy. (George, who had the scruffiest of shoes, the rattiest of pants, and the longest, wildest mane of reddish blond hair this side of the Serengeti, would in later years clean up good and make partner in a Philadelphia law firm.)

At the heart of the hippie movement, a current of activist concern ran deep. Although much of the movement was just fashion, indulgence, and predictable teen angst, a serious philosophy lay at its core. Vaguely articulated perhaps, but earnest.

It was about creating a revolutionary shift toward a better America with peace and love as its mantra—long before they became clichés. But since we didn't have any power, even if we'd wanted it, we rebelled as loudly as we could. I loaned my Fender Twin Reverb guitar amp as a speaker system at anti-war rallies at James Madison, and the rock band I was in included protest songs in its repertoire. We'd sing "Ohio," the Crosby, Stills, Nash, and Young lament about the four students killed by the National Guard at Kent State. We'd sing Country Joe McDonald's sarcastic "Fixin' to Die Rag," an anti-Vietnam War yowl telling the parents of America to "be the first one on the block to have your boy come home in a box." That we looked at all this through the lens of an adolescent mind was another matter entirely.

With more than a few nihilist and cynical strains, a restless mood was in the air of American culture. But the mood was also fed by a stream of fresh idealism, garnished with a dash of utopianism, that led to innovations like communes, food co-ops, and organic farming, to a new respect for the environment, and to a surge of interest in Eastern spirituality as well as natural methods of healing.

I loved the expressiveness and the exuberance that had been missing in my tight-lipped childhood and that was now being afforded by hippiedom. At one point, I had hair that fell past my shoulder blades—an imprimatur of rebellion and of a new value system. But my friends and I were cautious during those years in the Shenandoah Valley, as the more conservative folks there resented our long hair, occasionally throwing beer bottles at us, and even picking fights because of what our hair symbolized to them.

On more than one occasion, my friends and I were confronted in the dark or under the pale light of a lamppost by a group of young men brandishing chains and other steely tools of animosity. Only once did we get into a fight. I was sitting with three friends in the campus snack bar when a group of five young men from town walked in. After a few minutes, one of them came to stand next to me. Without a word, he punched me in the face. This set off a big brawl, and though I threw a few punches that didn't remotely make the whacking sounds they do in the movies, I was unhurt. But my roommate Larry was smacked hard on the head with a snack table.

When my band mates and I played rock and roll on stage, the soaring, feral abandon of it all was ecstatic. During our better moments, I found my cautious, hesitant self disappearing for a while. In that gap of time and space, when the constraints of my soul melted, I found rapture in flirting with the psychedelic muses. The bright exploding notes of song thrilled us, giving us a rush of new blood, hormones, and spirit. Whenever our performance hit the sweet spot and we played as one, all five of us felt electrified.

The Woodstock generation loved to blare its music at deafening levels, and though subsequent generations have maintained those volumes, this was new in stage performance. It was not just a boost to acetylcholine, serotonin, and endorphins. It was grace from the music demigods who, when satisfied that we'd met their criteria, would reach down not just with a finger but a whole fist.

The sweet paroxysm of those experiences made academic work seem insipid by comparison, a view reflected in my cumulative 1.8 grade point average, followed by academic probation, at the end of my junior year. Another emblem of this sort of vitality can be found in the grainy footage of teenage girls going hysterical at a Beatles concert. Their screaming, crying, and epileptic trembling were the joining of the Apollonian and Dionysian, of the innocent and the oh-so-slightly naughty, all blended to just the right combustible degree hot enough to make the heavens open up for them and to melt their little hearts. It was that sense of unbridled possibility that hung in the air in the late sixties and early seventies, weaving itself through the peaceful half-million at Woodstock and elsewhere in the country, suggesting a new dream for the ongoing social experiment of American culture. We found hints of the new dream in this wild new music that our parents detested—music that often left us high, though we were occasionally high in other ways too.

When I went to Sri Lanka, I immersed myself in the polar opposite of rock music's wilderness and its counterculture anthems. But the inward drift into quiet, still places may not have been what I needed most. This was confirmed decades later, when the pressure insisted that I stay active and expressive during the long-term task of cracking the shell built up around my soul. In the years since, the pressure has guided me, and taught me greatly about health, healing, and my unfinished work in the unconscious— self-knowledge that is now present every day in my work with my patients. But the message was clear: stay out of the monastery and find your place in conventional society.

In retrospect, it's clear that I became too enamored of beautiful meditative states before moving patiently through the earlier stages of ego development. Grasping at the highest rungs of the ladder, I ignored the lower rungs of development, as did some of my other contemporaries who belly-flopped into spiritual work early in life. What I had needed was to be socially normal and get a decent career going first as a foundation for my growth. Not that this pattern of growth applies to everyone, but for me personally, it was necessary. An idea from contemporary philosopher Ken Wilber not only illustrates the confusion that characterized my choices in those years, but provides a backdrop essential for understanding health as transformation and medicine as catalyst. I'll present it simplified.

States and stages: a crucial difference

In this concept from Wilber, a *state* is a particular condition at any given moment, such as when we're happy, sad, tired, or energetic. A stage, on the other hand, is a level of development. For example, our intelligence and maturity as wise elders reflect a stage of development more advanced than that of our teen years. Though we might be in similar states such as sadness or joy, we're at different stages. As we get older, we're nothing like our two-year-old selves. Similarly, a mature oak looks nothing like the seed from which it grew. Stages are permanent steps, while states come and go like clouds.

Once we've reached a stage of development, we are more complex and capable than before, and notably, we don't regress. For example, in college you don't need to relearn the lessons of high school. College doesn't negate high school, but instead stands on its shoulders. Once you've matured emotionally, you don't regress to the immaturity of a child. For the most part. With the human body, it's a little different, as in the very end—well, we know what happens. But we can nevertheless keep advancing through the different stages of physical wellness and psychological or spiritual growth.

We can be at an unhealthy stage of health characterized by stress and inflammation, but in a positive feeling state from two strong cups of coffee, a few cigarettes, and compliments from the boss. Improving the state artificially doesn't help us advance to the next stage.

Conversely, we may have grown into the stage of a wise, insightful elder, but be in a state of grief from the death of a husband. At the same time, a teenager, at an early stage of development, may be grieving her breakup with a boyfriend.

Both she and the elder are in a *state* of grief, but they are at entirely different *stages* of their development. A person can feel a *state* of euphoria from heroin or cocaine, but be at a very early *stage* of biological or emotional development. Anyone at an early stage of social development, feeling shy and unsure, can be in a state of confidence and bluster after a few beers and a few puffs of marijuana.

We can be robust at an advanced stage of fitness, but temporarily in a terrible state with a bad cold. Examples of the movement through stages includes the growth of a puppy into a dog, a seed into a rose bush, or a small group of people into a large, complex organization.

A progressive effect

Aside from the remedial work needed in acute medical care, the essential thrust of medicine should be catalytic in nature and dedicated to promoting our growth through the stages—whether psychological, physical, or spiritual. Otherwise, we run the risk of having medicine, either conventional or holistic, simply help patients change from an unpleasant state to a pleasant one. This can have as progressive an effect as moving up and down on a playground seesaw. In contrast, the ideal is development toward self-actualization, toward becoming a wholly integrated human. This is a radical departure from how we normally think of the role of medicine.

Incidentally, it also happens to be a big departure from the philosophy of much of integrative medicine, or CAM. In many of these fields, such as massage, functional medicine, herbalism, nutrition counseling, the manipulative therapies like osteopathic manipulation and chiropractic, and in some approaches to acupuncture, the emphasis is still often on the state versus the stage of the body's health, and not on developmental growth.

A broader purpose for medicine

In philosophy, the search for metaphysical purpose is an important theme. In science, it is not; in fact, it is often thought irrelevant or naïve. It's certainly not measurable. But ultimately, the bedrock of science and this search for meaning are compatible. We can be awed equally by the great songs of destiny and by the mitochondria's magic in creating fuel for the body. The marriage of scientific objectivism to the soul of art, philosophy, and spirituality has been underway for decades now, though it's really a reconciliation since they were divorced only in the last couple of centuries.

A revolution in our approach to health and our healthcare system will occur when this reconciliation happens. Then a symptom will not be merely physical, nor will it be a meaningless, random event or an opponent to vanquish.

Instead, it will be seen as part of the evolutionary impulse thrusting against our inertia and our resistance, shoving us with strong but gentle hands toward the fullest expression of human possibility. The symptom is related, through and through, to the spiritual imperatives flowing in our veins. It represents our family ties to the spirits of nature. It's woven into the challenges of reclaiming our birthright of growing into a happy, fulfilled, healthy self.

A healthcare system that appreciates the intelligent role of our symptoms in the schematics of nature will help us grow in this regard. Sadly, we are wasting billions of dollars on healthcare aimed at symptoms that are only encouraging us to love more, hate less, relax more, drink less, sleep more, exercise, and eat our vegetables just like Mom said. The country spends a big percentage of its budget on the repetitive, unproductive cycle of repairing broken windows—time and time again, year after year. We need instead to develop public policy and economic incentives that feed the roots of wellness. Doing this will be a whale of a task, but at the least, it's a conceptual starting point. The system at large will change when the corporate world can make gargantuan amounts of money by keeping people healthy, vibrant, and out of the hospital. Right now, hospitals, as well as the entire pharmaceutical and medical equipment industries, profit only when people are sick. This is a fundamental flaw in design.

Health professionals in the clinic can exercise skills that evoke the same catalytic power that spring grants the rolling hillsides of oak and dogwood and sweet gum. When necessary, the patient can be repaired, as broken branches should be pruned. But as appropriate, health professionals can also help invigorate the patient's potential to live a vibrant life.

The ancient healing traditions knew that medicine, art, spirituality, diet, and exercise all had to be woven into a single cloth for healing. In those times, health was not the sole province of the body. As one example, the word yoga is Sanskrit for union with the divine. While this approach to health has become popular and even chic today, it originally intended for the well-honed body to be a stepping-stone for spiritual development, a physical floorboard for building the spirit. It included diet, meditation, the study of ancient scripture, and a relationship with a teacher. In another example, Tibetan medicine is practiced not just for healing an individual patient, but for the sake of all beings. Its ultimate purpose is to help people achieve a final freedom from earthly suffering.

In integrative medicine, we can enfold the conversations of science into the understanding that, in the end, the real work is to help people reach their highest potential. We would help push this forward by insinuating the ethos of art and poetry into the semiconscious daze that permeates much of our culture and our schooling. A fusion of art, science, and morals into a new integral vision of health will ideally be both cause and attribute of medicine's transformation.

The arts are flesh and science is bone: science needs art and morals—the poetry, spark, and bluster—to find its true place in the world. With regard to health, the artistic self needs science. The unbound aesthetic self can fly off on the balloons of fancy, and the itchy lust for creativity can ignore the value of hard thinking, of logic and reason, of screwing nuts onto bolts. In an integrative world, all these necessary pieces of the puzzle can fit together neatly into a single whole—with medicine as catalyst and health as transformation.

Chapter Five

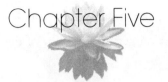

The Courage to Heal

I once asked a patient, "Are you a woman or a mouse?" Fortunately, she laughed. I'd been treating her for nearly twenty years, so our friendship allowed the teasing. Although she needed to be resolute in the legal and emotional circus of her divorce, she was wobbling from the fear of her ex-husband's wrath. She was losing sleep, feeling stressed, becoming fatigued, and dealing with it all with the pharmacological intervention of red wine. She could have cushioned her stress with massages, acupuncture, medications, or more merlot, but her core health issue was the need to act boldly. Whether she used natural or pharmacological methods to blunt her fear wasn't the point. What we needed was the right diagnosis and the right remedy.

For her insomnia, fatigue, and stress, the diagnosis was fear and the remedy courage. While the acupuncture treatments helped her feel relaxed and mentally clearer, these effects are better seen as a beginning, not the end. Ideally, the next step would be for her to use the clarity and relaxation as starting blocks, for rousing her innate strengths, and then acting courageously.

The physical symptoms were pointing directly at this need for courage. Whether she used an herb or a medication, she risked having the symptoms worsen unless she dug up their roots. In this case, as with most, strategy mattered far more than tactics. She would do better by resisting the seduction of a quick fix, which ultimately wouldn't be a fix anyway, and by plunging headfirst into her fear. A treatment that would only help her relax would be the repair of a broken window. Relaxation is not always the best antidote for stress. Instead, insight followed by effective action gets to the heart of the matter.

What I wanted for her was to become strong, not relaxed—relaxation would be the byproduct. Her state of tension, stress, and anxiety was different from her need to advance to the next stage of development, which was to find her primal courage. Any method or substance—whether valerian root or a sleeping pill—would be best used if it supported her in cooperating with the messages contained in her stress.

> Courage is the price that Life exacts for granting peace.
>
> —Amelia Earhart

In this case, the impulses of growth were encouraging her to be a woman and not a mouse. If this pushing were blocked, numbed, or tucked away in denial, she would delay the strengthening of her character. The stridency of her stress was the very fuel propelling her growth. This step-by-step slogging through the muck is endemic on the hero's journey. Why take that away from her? The well-intended efforts of professionals to help her relax could postpone that queasy moment when she would whirl around, take a stand, and reclaim her audacity.

Although courage and health are rarely mentioned in the same breath, and although they seem an odd couple, they go together well. When we think of health, we usually see pictures of fruit, vegetables, spas, and a slim athlete leaping through the air—not the many faces of the soul and spirit. But these elements of the human experience—courage and fear, love and rage, ecstasy and grief—reside in the landscape of our skin, nerves, arteries, and organs and cannot be ignored.

In fact, the idea that courage is an ingredient of health was a major motivation for me to write this book in the first place. I have too often seen the unhealthy physical and emotional consequences resulting from the fear of standing up, of asserting our authentic selves, and from choosing to suffocate in polite silence. In the treatment room, peeling off layers of symptoms and illness often uncovers that fear—ranging from a nagging reluctance to exercise to the terror of being raped again. Courage is then often necessary in becoming and staying healthy. Vegetables and fruit, yes. Exercise, yes. And now, courage.

Courage, fear, and health

Matters of human character have traditionally belonged to moral, literary, and philosophical discourse. And the matter of health has lately belonged only to science. But today, the integrative model of health begins to dissolve the boundaries between them all. To understand this better, we might imagine that the mind resides in the cell, affecting cell function just as food and exercise do.

To heal, we may be called to push through the resistance in our limbs. To thrive, to absorb the gusto in wind, water, sun, and earth, we need to make sacrifices now and then. This is not to elevate suffering to an art, nor to advocate a masochistic or spartan aesthetic. That would be an extreme interpretation of the message, as comforts of the flesh, in the right measure and context, are healthy. But when our fixation on comfort brings inertia to the soul and rust to the limbs, that's a different story. From my years of clinical observations, I believe that this fixation lies behind a good deal of our illnesses and symptoms today.

Constraint by fear is unhealthy. The refusal, or even the hesitation, to do what's right for our growth and our physical wellbeing can be costly. As we've seen from the patient stories I've told, our symptoms are often asking us to purge our bodies of grief, resentment, fear, and sometimes, plain boredom. At other times, they ask that we take a chance, speak out and risk being unloved, or that we forgive and start loving even in the face of heartbreaking injustice. They often ask us to reject the entropy that follows the lust for security and fear of risk. They always demand what's best for us. Sometimes, all they ask is for us to eat an apple instead of a cookie or to get off the couch and go for a walk.

Fear stops the power and vitality lying in our veins. Whether it's the anxiety of confessing to past infidelities, of volunteering to take the huge assignment at work, of telling your mother you love and forgive her, of giving full voice to your grief, of taking a break from a frenetic pace, fear leads to coagulation of the life force. This prevents us from feeling existentially free, and therefore, from being healthier. Fear also desensitizes the body. It hampers our ability to acknowledge the truth, as denial is a cushion that helps us delay effective action.

As I give patients free rein to speak in the treatment room, the drift of our dialogue most often moves away from the physical symptoms that brought them to me in the first place. The natural course of the conversation then starts to reveal a textured, layered storyline of a unique life saturated with the sugar and salt of love and fear, stoked by the yearning for the freedom that comes when the thirst of the soul is slaked. The truths behind the symptom want to be heard—you can sense it in the treatment room like some unseen gnome or nymph with a life of its own, pressing outward from deep inside, hoping to emerge on full display. The diagnosis at the bottom of the other diagnoses is often hesitancy, anxiety, inertia, the suspension in the airless gap between desire and fear. The antidote is courage.

Kinds of courage

The courage needed to become and remain healthy takes a variety of shapes. One is the simple effort to break free of the inertia brought to us by what I'll call a culture of indulgence. While it may be an overstatement to use the word "courage" to describe the antidote to this inertia, it does take initiative to break the habits of our creature comforts when they're making us unhealthy.

The other shapes of courage include the hard work of looking inward and learning to be our authentic selves and unloading the burdens of unfinished emotional business, both of which we explored in the previous chapter. But before going further, here's a look at the role of culture in shaping our values and beliefs and therefore our health.

A culture of indulgence

In a world with an embarrassing wealth of indulgences available to those with even average incomes, it's easy to think that contentment comes from having it all and doing it all. The message in the air is to buy this and buy that, after which you'll have your piece of nirvana. In this wired world, we have unprecedented speed, control, and choice. Just a few decades ago, the scope of information, services, and products now at our fingertips was the stuff of science fiction.

Today, we can use the web to order goods directly from India or China with a credit card and have them on our doorsteps in a few days. A few clicks of a button, and in seconds, we have new music on the computer, paid for instantly through our online bank account. Another few clicks, and you'll find the best prices in the country for a book or a blender. With one click, five hundred or even a couple of thousand friends in your online social network will know of your latest adventures.

Creature comforts can certainly contribute to a healthy and fulfilling life. But when we're saturated by them, we risk falling under their spell. Severe and persistent stress hurts the brain and the body, while relaxing on a beautiful beach, getting a massage, or laughing during a comedy show can all help us feel healthier. For those who can afford a few days at a spa, getting deeply relaxed is a treat for mind and body. Massage can increase the production of endorphins, a morphine-like substance that leads to a sense of wellbeing and even euphoria, and the production of oxytocin, which is involved in the warmth of bonding with others and is abundant between mother and child.

Conversely, a life of hardship and deprivation is abrasive to the body, a premise supported by research indicating that poverty is strongly correlated with poor health and a shorter life. In fact, some research indicates that poverty is more strongly associated with poor health and a shortened life than any other influence, including poor nutrition and the lack of exercise. So sensual delight has its place. Compared to the brutal lives of our frontier forebears, those of us in wealthier countries are fortunate today to have these luxuries help us stay healthy.

But that's different from the sense of entitlement (not in its political sense) that can come from living in a culture of indulgence, and which affects the middle classes as well as the wealthy. Unfortunately, that entitlement is a distortion of the evolutionary drive toward security and happiness. The two are different in the way overeating is different from eating. The fitting role of pleasure and relaxation in a healthy life is one thing, but overindulgence that impairs health is another. The issue here is how we use pleasure and indulgences, not whether they're inherently good or harmful.

A gratuitous attachment to comfort can lead to a limp spirit. Watching a sitcom with beer and chips in hand doesn't inspire us to lead our best lives, or to seek the heights of human possibility, or at the least, to go for a walk. A culture of indulgence breeds inertia, a dependence on comfort and the endless pursuit of the delights available to the eyes, ears, nose, tongue, and skin. But at what cost? A bit of our aliveness and humanness. Or often, a lot of it. While the quality of life in a country generally improves in correlation with its wealth, the ensuing comfort may come with the price tag of a torpid life and a diminished life force. A recent report predicts that if the trend for diabetes in the U.S. continues to increase at the current pace, one in three of us will be diabetic by the year 2050.

At times, we are seduced, then kidnapped, by our fondness for comfort. But still we want to be healthier. As in Saturday morning cartoons from long ago, we have an angel on one shoulder and a devil on the other, one whispering, "Listen to me. Exercise and eat vegetables" and the other saying, "Don't pay attention to her. Watch TV and eat popcorn."

St. Augustine captured the essence of this dilemma when he reportedly wrote, "Lord, make me chaste. But not yet." We already know how to be fit and healthy, but we're often short on motivation. In rich countries, the expectations for a life of ease have become embedded in the background of our thinking as part of the paradigm, and paradigms are invisible.

A friend who is a nurse and director of a hospital's operation rooms lost sixty pounds over several years. It took not only a nutrition makeover with a big reduction in carbohydrates and processed foods, but a rigorous exercise regimen on top of a long work week. This included being at the gym by five in the morning, seven days a week. She continues with this schedule today. This woman has courage.

Another element of the idea of an indulgent culture is the overreliance on others for our health—or to put it more bluntly, the abdication of responsibility. That's different from the appropriate reliance on experts for medical concerns. We've been hearing for years about the importance of taking responsibility for our health, but that doesn't mean diagnosing ourselves or neglecting essential health care. But when we suffer from the harmful effects of an overindulgent life, only to rely on a doctor or other health professional to heal us, something's amiss. The fix-it model of healing we discussed earlier includes the expectation that someone else should fix me.

To be clear, I'll repeat that overreliance on others does not mean avoiding appropriate medical care when necessary. Instead, it refers to a value system that hasn't found merit in proactively engaging in our health and personal development. It's ironic to ask someone else to repair the damage after our health degenerates from an indulgent or abusive lifestyle.

Hidden messages

To further explore the role of culture in shaping our perspectives on health, a brief description of a concept put forth by linguist and author Deborah Tannen will help. In her books, Tannen has written books about the crucial role of implied messages that occur regularly in conversation. These hidden communications are called meta-messages. Their meaning is conveyed through nuanced insinuation, not explicitly in the spoken or written word. For example, the question, "Why'd you do that?" is, literally interpreted, just a request for information. But, in American idiom, it implies disapproval, so the listener is likely to feel guilty or offended by the question. And "It's OK, I'll do it myself" in many contexts can be a subtle, aggressive attempt to induce guilt.

Questions like "Are you going to order dessert again tonight?" or "You're wearing that?" (the title of one of her books) are full of innuendo. "Honey, we don't communicate well" is really an accusation that has sent a chill of anxiety through many a husband's spine. The real message is disguised by the words spoken.

We can then extrapolate this idea of a meta-message to the larger stage of culture and to the way values and beliefs are subtly disseminated. In the media, for example, values and norms are conveyed implicitly. When we see commercials for clothes or cars or the latest perfume, the meta-message includes standards and expectations about the good life as well as an entire value system framed by marketing tools and strategies. Nowhere in these ads do we find the meta-message that we're lucky to have a car that runs at all or to own an old CD player instead of the latest digital gadget. The implied suggestion is that we ought to have the best, the most, the newest. No one needs to say outright that you should live a life of indulgence. The message is conveyed powerfully enough by implication.

After years of clinical observations, it seems to me that the most common proximal sources of inertia are the allure of the sugar fairy, the siren call of daily drink, and the gravitational pull of the American couch. For many others, the inertia in taking care of their health comes from being under the whip of constant overwork and a frenzied schedule. They choose a lifestyle that allows them insufficient time to do good things for their bodies. These habits, which are at once cultural, psychological, and biochemical, help keep earthbound those who would otherwise fly.

I'm belaboring this point because the reinvention of health and healing needs us to think harder and to think bigger, and to see how culture shapes perceptions and expectations that directly influence our health, and by extension, the healthcare crisis. If the drift of our cultural norms has us thinking it's standard to sit in front of the TV with beer and pizza or chips and soda, then this soporific and hypnotic state holds our health hostage. It leads to the invention, in places like the Texas and Iowa state fairs, of deep-fried butter, deep-fried candy bars, and deep-fried Twinkies.

Our picture of the good life also includes the myth that happiness is the freedom to indulge without limits, an idea that, in part, shapes our prevailing model of retirement. Once we have enough money and time, then we'll do whatever we want—and then we'll be happy. But this isn't happiness any more than good parenting is letting your children do anything they want. The American Dream needs reinvention, and, in particular, the emblematic cornerstone of life, liberty, and the pursuit of happiness that informs this dream needs clarification.

Our animal instincts are based in the limbic system of the brain, and when it's given free rein, it wants what it wants, when it wants, how it wants. But the prefrontal cortex, which is the part of the brain governing rational and executive functions, will usually kick in when fully developed to help us temper these primitive urges. It recognizes that the primal energies of the animal self, however necessary for the verve and hustle we need to live a robust life, must have a counterweight in the rational self. This idea is not new. It saturates film, theatre, literature, psychology, and the spiritual traditions. The American Dream, however much it needs to be redefined, was never about self-indulgence in the first place.

Courage may not be the best word for what we need to escape this orbit of overindulgence. We might call it chutzpah, panache, nerve, or gumption. But we need something of the sort for overcoming inertia and for sustaining optimal health and vitality. Certainly, life can unfold effortlessly at times in astonishing flow and synchronicity. But as star athletes and musicians say, those moments of flow graced by a magical unfolding of events come only to those who were first disciplined enough to put great effort into their art. Michael Jordan practiced more than did any of his teammates. Ted Williams would go home in the evening after team practice and continue practicing his swing until his hands sometimes bled.

It takes a little sweat equity to escape the drift of an indulgent culture—an idea echoed in Edison's saying that genius is 99 percent perspiration. On the other hand, many people have created lifestyles that are healthy and enjoyable without much discipline. But my perspective on this comes from observing the average American for decades now and seeing the common denominators: there are constant challenges in designing a lifestyle that works. In most cases, doing the right thing requires at least a little effort.

The first type of courage, then, confronts sluggishness and inertia, and leads to sweating on the treadmill, running a 10K, kayaking on the river, playing tennis, and retraining the taste buds to go for the crispness of vegetables and the charm of fruit instead of being seduced by foods fabricated in factories.

As we look further into these ideas, we find other kinds of courage.

The courage to grieve

"I've been trying to be strong," said Alma. Since the death of her husband two months earlier, she'd been containing her tears. She'd been married to him for over fifty years and had hardly spent a day apart from him since they met in their teens. In her words, she was trying not to be weak. And crying signified weakness. Sturdy women, especially in the fishing town where they'd lived, could tough it out with their heads up just like the men. Since the strong bones and big muscles of watermen were a hallmark of their culture, the women too needed to show pioneer strength. However, a back problem she'd had in the past became excruciating after her husband died. She was desperate, especially since medications and steroid injections hadn't helped.

On the morning following her first acupuncture treatment, she woke up to notice that her back pain was almost gone. Then, without warning, she cried for three solid hours over the death of her husband in a discharge of bottled-up grief. Over the following months, she learned to make friends with that grief, and slowly both her grief and her back pain began to subside. During that time, we spoke almost exclusively about her emotions, not about her back pain, which eventually seemed incidental to both of us. She saw how her back pain increased whenever she was sad or lonely. She saw how the mind and body communicated with each other: the moods worsened her pain and the pain worsened her moods. She came to recognize the symptom as a message; she knew it was instructing her to grieve fully, to stop isolating herself, to welcome the support being offered by friends and family. She saw how the courage to embrace her grief, not the ability to push it aside, was the true test of her strength. Eventually, her back pain decreased considerably and she was able to move on with her life.

Grieving takes courage. It's a knife-edge in the soul, likely to make the hardiest among us gasp for our spiritual breath, and often for our physical breath. But it must have its day. It will insist. When denied, no matter how unjust its cause, it can seep into blood, muscle, joints, and organs. It's resolute, heaving against the walls of denial and resistance until its needs are met or reduced to a fraction of their original intensity. The body demands completion and resolution because it can't withstand a lifetime of grief. Shakespeare wrote of the need to put our grief into words:

> *Give sorrow words.*
> *The grief that does not speak,*
> *whispers the o'erfraught heart*
> *and bids it break.*

While our loss may seem unjust when those who have died were young or were victimized, the steadfastness of the healing impulse demands resolution nevertheless. It is surprisingly obstinate, insisting that we resolve this, heal that, complete this. Day after day, it nudges and prods us to make compost of our unfinished emotions. We may need years of grueling inner work before the loss no longer brings us to our knees. We may need to expunge loneliness, self-pity, rage, bitterness, a sense of guilt, remorse, or injustice—all of which can follow the death of a loved one, and none of which are grief itself, but its accoutrements. In time, and in imperceptible measure, the grief may soften and come passing by on fewer occasions like a gray cloud that appears for a while and then moves on for the day. To this point, George Eliot wrote:

*She was no longer wrestling with the grief, but could sit down with it
as a lasting companion and make it a sharer in her thoughts.*

One illustration of emotion's impact on the body is a condition known
as stress cardiomyopathy, or Tako-Tsubo cardiomyopathy. More simply, it's
called broken-heart syndrome. First identified in the early 1990s and now
more widely accepted in cardiology than at first, the condition mimics a heart
attack. It has the usual sensations and appearances of a heart attack, such
as severe chest pains, but shows no evidence of such through the standard
medical tests.

The reason for this is that the broken-heart syndrome is triggered by
severe emotional or physical stress and is not a real heart attack. In 2004, a
tour boat in the Inner Harbor of Baltimore capsized during an unexpected
storm. A twenty-six-year-old woman and her boyfriend were among those
who drowned. Though her parents were also in the boat, they survived.
Later that night, the mother had what appeared to be a heart attack and was
admitted to the coronary care unit at Johns Hopkins. But after conducting
the usual tests, her doctors found that she hadn't had a true heart attack, but
rather stress cardiomyopathy. Her heart had been stunned and overwhelmed
by the surge of stress hormones that flooded her body, the handprints of the
unbearable pain that followed the death of her child.

For centuries, both Chinese and Indian medicine have claimed that
the heart is conscious and is the seat of love. Acupuncture points related to
the heart include Spirit Gate, Spirit Path, and Utmost Source, a nod to this
relationship between the heart and consciousness. In the West, we've spoken
for centuries of the warm heart, cold heart, broken heart, heart of stone, heart
of gold. In the Bible, King Solomon said, "A merry heart doth good like
medicine." Again from Shakespeare, "A light heart lives long."

In recent years, the field of neurocardiology was created after researchers found evidence that the heart has, in essence, a mini-brain of its own. The heart has neurons—yes, that's brain cells in the heart—that let it react independently of the brain in emotional responses. This in turn affects heart function—a process clearly involved in the broken heart syndrome. The image of a broken heart, capturing the essence of this mother's experience, is less metaphorical than we thought.

I have found in my clinical experience that both men and women are susceptible to the fallacy that the suppression of grief is a sign of strength. Perhaps it's partly cultural and partly the understandable, primal instinct to avoid pain. In any case, when grief is prevented from having its say, it will speak through the body. At the least, most people feel leaden and deflated during periods of grief. At worst, pain or some disorder may arise in the shoulder, back, skin, lungs, bowels—any part of the body is fair game.

When grief crosses the threshold from the realm of emotion into the body, the symptom feels remarkably physical—because it is. It isn't psychosomatic, a word often used to imply it isn't real. On the contrary, it's assuredly real since the patient truly hurts—a view that conveys a deep respect for the patient's subjective world even in the absence of measurable evidence. The symptom should be considered authentic, and, like all other symptoms, seen as a finger pointing to the moon. We just need to look and listen more closely. That grief or another emotion is manipulating tissue and cell to serve as loudspeakers doesn't render the symptom unreal.

One elderly retiree who came to me for shoulder pain had been grieving five years over the death of his wife. Lingering far longer than usual, his sorrow was as stark as if she'd died a month ago. As we discussed his life, he revealed that he was tormented by the guilt for having slept with several other women while he was married. He had never confessed his infidelity to his wife. Since she had died presuming his loyalty, he was tortured by a regret that complicated and prolonged his grief. Without closure, the grief was using his shoulder as a sounding board.

Whether grief comes from the loss of a loved one, childhood abuse, or any other trauma, it requires us to be fully conscious and receptive, to let it burn like wildfire through our souls. It needs to be heard, to be understood. After it has burned itself up, the soul is made bigger, stronger, and once again whole.

The courage to assert

Peggy came in one day to see me after a long absence. After her initial series of treatments a few years earlier, she had moved to a maintenance schedule of a treatment every month or two, but then hadn't kept up for some time. After she came in and sat down, she started telling me about the recent onset of some pain. But then she began to cry. Her husband had decided, without consulting her, to sell their waterfront estate. She loved the place, filled with memories of family gatherings with the grandchildren boating, swimming, and running about. But her husband had decided, on his own, to sell the house because it made sense financially. Since they were both getting older, he said, they should buy a smaller home and reduce the expenses of keeping up the house and grounds. As distraught as she was, Peggy was afraid to speak up and risk a verbal beating.

As we discussed this, she recognized that her stress came not only from the possible loss of her home, but from being a woman without a voice. After a couple of acupuncture treatments and further dialogue, she came in one day looking chipper. The acupuncture had reduced her pain, which led to her feeling a new clarity and energy, which in turn helped her become assertive enough to express herself to her husband. To her surprise, she'd been able to convince him to pull the house off the market. Contrary to what she had feared most, they were now getting along better than ever.

As the design of the mind demands that we feel whole, complete, and resolved, the courage to speak our truth helps create a sense of wholeness, which in turn is good for the flesh. When we are weighed down by anxious silence, by an encumbered soul, or by anything leaving us off kilter, the body carries a heavy load.

While growing up, most of us weren't taught how to resolve conflicts in relationship. We usually learned to suffer in silence, as inelegantly disgorging our anger rarely led to good results. Now with our adult—and rightful—notions of civility, we often choose to stay mute. But between these two extremes, we have the option of speaking directly, authentically, and kindly with the clear and definite intention to dissolve the conflict. When silence turns an intimate relationship frosty, the low temperatures can freeze the soul. This then leads to an imbalance in body chemistry.

While the gruff and drunken Norman Mailer isn't usually quoted in books on health and healing, he once made a noteworthy comment on the value of speaking up. He wrote that one of Tolstoy's recurring themes could be distilled as, "Compassion is valueless without severity, (otherwise it cannot defend itself against sentimentality)."

Although the message might sting, speaking our truth honors the listener. When speaking our truth, the meta-messages to the other person might include: you matter; I trust that you are mature enough and strong enough to bear the unpleasantness of my truth; you are not so capricious as to leave me over this incident; I know you love me enough to work with me on restoring our intimacy and trust.

Out of fear of hurting others or of being hurt, we may take politeness to an extreme. It then becomes only about preserving the peace, keeping the sentiments placated, which is as useful as letting a child do and buy anything he wants just to avoid upsetting him. When fear of the sting suffocates the expression of necessary truths, both parties suffer in the end. Of course, at the other extreme, a prolonged, rowdy skirmish of a relationship will also unhinge our blood chemistry.

In most countries, we don't fear for our lives when expressing our truth. But we do fear the death of our self-image, the death of rejection by those we love most, the death of humiliation, the capital punishment of not belonging. But if we speak authentically, then the life force in every cell is free to flow abundantly and keep our flesh healthy. Catharsis doesn't mean blurting out any emotion that comes to mind, nor does self-expression mean wanton criticism, name-calling, or plate throwing. Those are destructive extremes. But being courageous enough to speak effectively and honestly, which is to speak constructively, lightens the weight of body and soul. The courage to assert includes living with integrity, acting in concert with our deepest passions and highest principles, moving in lockstep with our truth. It just so happens to be good for the body.

The courage to be vulnerable

When Steve first came to see me, he was struggling with fatigue, indigestion, irritability, and a serious craving for sugar. To help with his fatigue, he would drink twelve cups of coffee daily, many sodas, and eat a surfeit of desserts. He might have been categorized as a dessertarian.

After two months of acupuncture treatments, his body was more energetic, the indigestion eliminated, his moods better. But during one session, he started to weep as he spoke of being alienated from several family members. The pain of rejection had been troubling him for years, but now, without the diversion of his physical symptoms, he was getting a taste of his bottled-up sadness.

In his case, eating mounds of desserts was serving not only to give his moods an immediate boost but also to numb the turmoil. Eating pastries and cookies and drinking fourteen sodas a week had been easier. The distractions caused by the disturbances in his blood chemistry had been serving a purpose. To admit to his feelings of vulnerability took courage, and as his healing moved forward, he was forced to confront the unresolved business of his life.

In many cases, healing is a far simpler affair. In 1983 at a conference in Washington, D.C., Yeshi Dhonden, the personal physician for the Dalai Lama for twenty years, said that sometimes a knee pain is just a knee pain. Legend has it that Freud once said sometimes a cigar is just a cigar. Some symptoms are just physical. But the physical body is an avatar for the spiritual self, and in many cases, our physical malaise is making the ambiguous, semiconscious doings of the soul more accessible to the conscious mind. Steve was being turned about to face the wisdom pressing itself into his life.

The courage to fling open the doors of the soul is often necessary for healing. The vulnerability that this entails is not weakness, but on the contrary, a reflection of true strength—a kind of strength markedly different from the domination and control we normally associate with power. Instead, it's the power that comes from sitting squarely in our truth, from being immersed in healing wisdom, as awful as it may be at times. If we choose to see it this way, grief is medicine.

The courage to risk

Barbara was a thoughtful, sensitive woman resigned to an unhappy life. She and her husband, who was uninterested in any dialogue about their marriage, lived in a cold limbo without having had sex in twelve years. Her husband refused to discuss their impasse or to go with her to a marriage counselor, believing that nothing was wrong and that there was nothing to discuss. Though she had originally come to see me for fatigue, stress, headaches, and joint pains, she was well aware that the tangled knots of her life were contributing to her symptoms. Fortunately, she began to feel happier as we proceeded in treatments, and the fatigue, stress, and pain decreased. But as she became more awake and aware, she came to what she hadn't wanted to admit: there was little hope for the marriage.

The stronger Barbara became, the more she realized that a happier life was possible. After many moments of trance-like euphoria from her acupuncture treatments, after feeling the vibrancy of joy spreading into her life, she had glimpses of what a fulfilling life might look like. But though she was able to laugh more often, she also felt saddened at the thought of dissolving her marriage. At least her vitality was on the move. When she'd been tired and stressed, the thought of risking a life on her own had been overwhelming. When she became stronger, she was able to take a few small steps toward independence.

As people become healthier, they become more animated. A fire comes to the eyes, a quickening to the hands, a liveliness to the voice. Most people who experience this believe it's from the absence of their pain or other symptoms, but my suspicion is that it's less linear than that. I see the relationship between symptoms and overall vitality as being similar to the relationship between the front and back of the hand. Or to put it another way, it's bidirectional: the symptom and overall energy feed each other in a chicken-or-egg cyclicality. The more emotional stress you feel, the worse your pain. The worse your pain, the more emotional stress. The happier you feel, the better your body will feel and the more likely you will be free of pain.

The price of health

Health, vibrancy, and resilience come at a price. The price might be sweating during a run, huffing on a bike, or crying unshed tears. Whatever form it takes, we are often called to push hard, and this effort can then give birth to new muscle, whether anatomical or spiritual. When people are in vibrant health, they've usually worked at achieving it. Whether you're thirty or eighty, the juices of regeneration are waiting in your flesh and bones.

A reasonable discipline in the face of seductive pleasures can go a long way. It takes nerve to resist the sweet singing voice of ice cream or the come-hither of succulent homemade chocolate chip cookies calling your name every night after dinner. Your belly brazenly says you must indulge, while your rational mind meekly says you shouldn't. Or maybe it's OK. Maybe just one scoop.... There are times to simply flow with the momentum, and then there are times to press against habit and to soundproof the freezer and cookie jar. At those times, the act of indulging is not evidence that you live a quality life or that you're being a free spirit. It's a mild form of addiction.

From my conversations with patients over the decades, it seems that it's this inertia that holds tight reins on our good intentions, an idleness that is now epidemic. One research study found Americans spending nine times as many minutes watching television and doing other leisurely activities than on exercise and all other physical activities combined.

The good news is that exercising regularly and eating well can eventually come easily and naturally. In the field of addictions treatment, white-knuckle sobriety is a label given to the early stages of abstinence in which the addict strains against the seductive invitation of just one drink. The cravings usually recede over time. Similarly, getting into the habits of good health may require some white-knuckling at first, but this can, and should, become effortless eventually. The body will want to be active, it will want fruit and vegetables, and it can become averse to processed foods. Fighting our urges too hard can lead to a backlash.

As we saw earlier, the hero's battle with hostile creatures on the road to self-actualization is the very stuff of growth. The fight helps the seeds of character sprout, making us more capable and more robust. We've seen that from a biochemical and metabolic point of view, stress is necessary. So it is with the psychological and spiritual journey.

If we cling to our resentments, if we fear standing up for ourselves, if we refuse to grieve as we must, if we deplete ourselves caring for others, our bodies will protest. They'll then assume the work of expressing what we've chosen to keep silent. But since they can't form words and sentences, they gesture with insomnia, headaches, a pain in the belly, an ache in the shoulder, a shroud of weariness—or a thousand other ways at the disposal of human physiology. If we ignore these attempts to change us—whether through denial, fear, suppression, food, alcohol, or drugs—they'll send progressively louder signals until they reach deafening volumes. The courage to feel the pain in our souls is necessary in having a resilient, vibrant body. Living irresolute has its costs.

Our greatest fears lie in the shadowy parts of the soul where we store grief, humiliation, terror, or rage—none of which will dissolve when ignored. While it may take as much boldness to make certain decisions in careers or relationships as to ski off a cliff, an even greater courage is needed to open the soul wide, to become vulnerable enough to scrape out emotional detritus. For some people, it may be news to learn of this unfinished business. Others are simply reluctant, understandably, to do the hard work.

Barbara, whom we met earlier, was also concerned about the loss of her dearest friendship after a conflict about eight years earlier. The apparent rejection by this close female friend left her with lingering remorse. As we talked, she recognized that she was afraid of possible rejection if she reached out. The relationship had ended oddly, abruptly, and Barbara didn't know why. After deciding to find her friend, she found the contact information through a web search, and the two used email to set a time to talk over the phone. During the week before the scheduled call, Barbara became highly agitated, unable to sleep more than a few hours at night. She worried about all that could go wrong and about possibly being hurt again. Given the closeness of their friendship in the past, she found the thought of rejection unbearable.

Finally, she spoke with her friend, who, as it turned out, had been equally puzzled and saddened by the loss of their friendship. When they found out how much each had missed the other, their relationship was instantly made whole. They were ecstatic, vowing to never let it happen again. For days afterward, Barbara was euphoric. Over the following weeks, she was better able to stick with her goals for exercising and for eating healthily—which in turn increased her energy further. Barbara's willingness to do some housecleaning in the dusty corners of her past was a major influence in this jump forward in her overall physical health. As Anaïs Nin wrote, "Life shrinks or expands in proportion to one's courage."

Food as sedative

Fear persuades us to find many ways of avoiding the rough edges that often characterize the impulse to grow. Food is one of them. In 2003, Louise Dallman, Ph.D., and her team at UCLA published groundbreaking research that showed how we can sedate ourselves naturally with food. For the first time, we had a study demonstrating the scientific basis of comfort eating.

In their experiment, laboratory rats were fed high-calorie foods, such as those laden with fat, sugar, and simple carbs. The study showed how the rats' metabolism reacted by signaling the hypothalamic-pituitary-adrenal axis (HPA) to slow down the production of cortisol from the adrenal glands. Cortisol and epinephrine (or adrenaline) are the two key stress hormones—the jittery ones.

We've long suspected that people overeat to comfort themselves, but here was the physiological map laid out for the first time. It explained how we can induce pharmacological sedation with large amounts of cookies, cakes, pasta, pizzas, chocolate, candy, fast food, bread, or french fries. That rich creamy German chocolate cake with a big dollop of vanilla ice cream is literally a tranquillizer.

Dallman's study also found that contrary to previous opinion, body fat is not an inert substance. Instead, it is to a degree like an extra endocrine gland that sends messages to the HPA axis just as dietary sugar and fat do to reduce cortisol production. This suggests that extra padding on the body helps keep us calm, though at a high price.

Referring to what I've written so far about the symptom's strategy, we can now redefine overeating as a symptom: a well-intended but injurious attempt by the body and mind to find balance. The imbalance is set off by nervousness, tension, sadness, resentment, or any emotion that makes the body restless or otherwise uncomfortable. But instead of grappling with the problem, we can block it out by eating, just as we might obstruct sunlight with a window shade.

When blood sugar is repeatedly spiked by a big infusion of simple carbs, and then lowered by insulin secreted from the pancreas, it can become habitually low. This in turn can lead to food cravings we can't foil just by pursing our lips. After exposure to repeated deluges of blood sugar over the years, the body can then become insulin resistant—a condition where it can't absorb any more sugar.

When blood sugar can no longer be shunted into the cells by insulin, it has nowhere to go. It stays in the bloodstream, leading to elevated blood sugar, a pre-diabetic condition. Then without a change in dietary habits, it can lead to full blown diabetes over time.

But a purely scientific view of diabetes or any disease obscures the human comedy, or tragedy, woven into the storyline of our cells, blood, and hormones. The impact of divorce, an adult son on drugs, or fatigue from caring for a mother with dementia—all can distort blood chemistry. Diabetics often find their blood sugar rising after becoming angry, stressed, or depressed.

This is where an integrative approach to medicine can provide an invaluable new perspective for those trying to become and stay healthy. It suggests that diabetes or any other disease is usually about more than what's measured by diagnostic tests. It's about the call to grow and transform, to make the best of our talents for living a fulfilling life.

If we look at health as transformation, and medicine as a catalyst for that transformation, then every symptom, struggle, or disease can be seen as an opportunity to learn and grow. They may be painful, or even excruciating, but they can be the next step in our growth if we so choose. What's needed for our growth may be as simple as outwitting the culture of indulgence, or as difficult as calling forth the greatest courage we've ever had to muster.

A quick review

In tying this all together, a review of all we've covered so far may help. We started with the idea from Chapter Two that the symptom is a message.

Then in Chapter Three, we examined the idea that this message comes from the extraordinary wellspring of healing in both body and mind.

In Chapter Four, we saw how the message is often not just a repair order, but the demand of the evolutionary impulse that we develop into the best and healthiest individual we can be. If we are to transform, we need to face the obstacles on the path: lethargy, fear, resentment, narcissism, and so on, and transcend them. Medicine, redefined, can be a catalyst for this change.

Now in this chapter, we've seen how we need courage to respond to the tribunals of physical, psychological, or spiritual growth. It's an element of our physical health.

This picture is radically different from the prevailing view of health and healing we find in both the media and scientific circles, and even in a large swath of holistic medicine. It infers that under all the layers of the personal human drama, after all the tests and diagnoses, we often find that one of the requisites of healing may be courage—for our own sake as well as that of our loved ones and our world.

Chapter Six

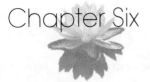

Meaning, Purpose, and Health

In February 2006, in the Hudson Bay village of Ivujivik, a forty-one-year-old Inuit woman was walking in front of her seven-year-old son when she turned around to see a polar bear getting ready to attack the boy. With no other option in sight, the woman charged the bear and began beating on it with her fists. The seven-hundred-pound bear knocked her down twice—which means, it should be noted, that she kept getting back up. In short order, a hunter in the village came and shot the bear.

After reading this story in a Washington Post article, I asked myself, "Under what circumstances would I attack, with my bare hands, a hungry seven-hundred-pound, eight-foot tall behemoth of bone-crunching muscle with sharp claws and jagged teeth?" Very few, and loved ones in danger comes to mind. The raw vitality that surged through this mother's arms came from her unequivocal purpose—she was ready to risk mortal injury for the child she loved.

The story is one illustration of the way purpose and meaning can create energy, a point that rarely enters a discourse on health. Energy often rises to meet a demand, polar bear emergencies aside, and a meaningful purpose can have this sort of impact on our lives as a whole. I'd like to explore this idea in two of its aspects: the first is the immediate and momentary impact of meaning and purpose on our vitality as we saw in the story of the Inuit woman. The second is its more diffuse effect on our health and on our lives as a whole.

Health for...

In an earlier chapter, I wrote that we want health for a purpose, not just for its own sake. We want health in *order to*: follow our dreams, work and play, love people. Unless we've just recovered from an illness, we don't bask in sitting around being healthy. Alone, it's not enough for fulfillment. When we're sick, the restoration of health certainly becomes the Holy Grail, but once restored, it fades into the background like a passerby absorbed into a sidewalk crowd.

Health, like anything else, always occurs in context: it occurs in a body and mind that are part of a family living in a town in a country on a beautiful planet in a galaxy in a universe. Health is valuable to us *because*. When it's present, we don't notice it. Instead, we attend to the joy of riding bikes with our children, the satisfaction of a good day at work, the pleasure of hearing a beautiful aria.

Understanding health requires seeing how it fits into the big picture of our lives. We can never wholly understand it by peering into a microscope, however valuable and powerful the resulting data. Imagine trying to understand human nature by putting a man in a locked cell in a lab and closely watching his every move and every mood. We could watch him every second of the day from a dozen different camera angles, monitoring his heart rate, brain waves, and blood chemistry. But in this artificial context, we wouldn't understand the scope and depth of his humanness. That would only emerge in his interactions with other people and the world at large—in other words, in context—because human behavior is best understood at the crossroads between self and other. True, much can be learned from observing a man isolated in distressing conditions, but the picture will be distorted and grossly incomplete. A wolf in the zoo is not the creature it is in the wild.

Similarly, any snapshot we take of health—whether in the form of blood tests, MRIs, or the palpation of a knot in the shoulder—is a static picture of a dynamic process. The snapshot captures one moment from one angle that is frozen in time. It may be accurate, but it's also incomplete. In its full glory, health is a teeming, purring, multidimensional occasion—yes, an occasion—*that cannot have full identity apart from its context.* Health and disease aren't things; they're like the river of Heraclitus. Chinese medicine acknowledges this by saying that the organs of the body are processes like changing clouds.

This idea is again central to the story of the broken window, where multiple influences led to the symptom, and where we get the most accurate diagnosis by understanding the whole story. Health and disease then are best understood in relationship to something else: food, exercise, emotions, work, lifestyle, and so on. Context gives clarity to both illness and health.

In a larger context, health is influenced by meaning, purpose, and values. As vague as this might sound in a dialogue usually marked by concrete words like cells and organs, it is, in my view, profoundly related to the state of our health. Our health, without fail, occurs within the context shaped by our values, our sense of purpose, the meaning we give to our lives. Because our values and the resulting priorities fashion our activities, schedules, and lifestyles, they're a matrix of our health.

For instance, if a person's values lead her to drive obsessively and unhealthily toward her career goals, then the ensuing inflammation, high blood pressure, headaches, and aching muscles are meaningful only in the context of those values. I have had countless conversations with my patients in which they discover how their symptoms come from the contours of their lives, which in turn are shaped by their values and priorities.

We might find, for example, that the headaches and insomnia come from eating poorly and not exercising, which come from not having enough time, which comes from being too busy at work, which comes from the desire to have a certain income, which comes from priorities, which come from values shaped by the need for security in the financial hierarchies of society. When a person's value system leads to a lifestyle that leads to disease, the distorted value system is the primary diagnosis.

Meaning, purpose, and energy

As we saw from the story of the Inuit woman, energy can rise to meet an immediate demand in the moment. If our customer is waiting, we'll have a boost of energy to do our job even when tired. If we're about to walk on stage, we'll also get a boost of energy. A commitment to others in the performance of a task, whether it's to sell them shirts or make a presentation to the board of directors, calls forth a surge of vitality. But let's explore the way energy responds to less tangible and immediate demands.

> Many persons have a wrong idea of what constitutes true happiness. It is not attained through self-gratification but through fidelity to a worthy purpose.
>
> –Helen Keller

If you ask people what matters most to them, the answers are usually about making a difference in the lives of others. If we dig deep enough, we'll usually find altruistic inclinations, and people will usually tell you that, in the end, what matters most is other people. As there's often a difference between espoused values and behavior, people may not always act in accordance with these sensibilities. But when pressed by circumstances, like the Inuit woman, our best can come forth.

The tragedy of September 11 brought out a remarkable compassion and solidarity among New Yorkers. Natural disasters like the 2004 tsunami, the 2010 Haiti earthquake, the trapped miners of Chile in 2010, and the 2011 tsunami in Japan elicited a tremendous outpouring of sympathy and support from around the world. The need to care already existed, lying in wait to express itself, and instantly arose from the ashes of tragedy.

Meaning and purpose are not abstractions, but energy. They're what we wake up into in the morning, however distant they might be in the background as we climb out of our pajamas. They're not just charming ideas, obligatory moral stands, or feathers in our social caps, but more like an existential soup that lends its flavor to all the ingredients of our lives. They reshape us and reposition us in the world. Because a meaningful purpose is a form of energy, it contributes to health. As we further explore this idea, a few thoughts from the mystics will help.

Some mystics tell us that the world, or more accurately, the World, is seeking healing and integration through our individual hands, feet, and voices. In a simple and most elegant way, Martin Buber captured the idea when he wrote, "Unity is a not a property of the world, but its task." Purpose, in this sense, is not just a noble idea but an emblem of the world's search for unity among its disconnected parts.

This is similar, if not identical, to Brian Swimme's idea of allurement, a gravitational urge in the world encouraging unity between people and things. This allurement wants the world more whole, to have us heal the sick, to feed the hungry, to have nations at peace. What's noteworthy here, and most relevant to our discussion, is that when we are so aligned with this allurement, we have more energy in mind and body. It's as though the world rewards us when we support its mission. Nature's resources—whether we call them spirit, *qi*, or adenosine triphosphate—work in service of the world's evolutionary impulse for perpetuating itself, for growing and evolving as a planet and as the human race.

When Helen Keller wrote that happiness comes from fidelity to a worthy purpose, she echoed the sentiments of many thinkers throughout the centuries. We find another expression in Viktor Frankl, an Austrian neurologist and psychiatrist whose approach to therapy was shaped by three years in Auschwitz, Theresienstadt, and Turkheim near Dachau. He believed that a strong sense of meaning and purpose was necessary for health and survival, a belief that came from observing how inmates in the concentration camps seemed to have better chances of surviving if guided by a strong sense of purpose. From the insights that came through his work in supporting his fellow inmates, he created a new approach to therapy that he called logotherapy. In *Man's Search for Meaning*, he wrote:

> *Don't aim at success—the more you aim at it and make it a target, the more you are going to miss it. For success, like happiness, cannot be pursued; it must ensue...as the unintended side-effect of one's personal dedication to a course greater than oneself.*

In describing how he came to his conclusions, he writes elsewhere in the book:

> *We stumbled on in the darkness, over big stones and through large puddles, along the one road leading from the camp. The accompanying guards kept shouting at us and driving us with the butts of their rifles. Anyone with very sore feet supported himself on his neighbor's arm. Hardly a word was spoken; the icy wind did not encourage talk. Hiding his mouth behind his upturned collar, the man marching next to me whispered suddenly: "If our wives could see us now! I do hope they are better off in their camps and don't know what is happening to us."*
>
> *That brought thoughts of my own wife to mind. And as we stumbled on for miles, slipping on icy spots, supporting each other time and again, dragging one another up and onward, nothing was said, but we both knew: each of us was thinking of his wife. Occasionally I looked at the sky, where the stars were fading and the pink light of the morning was beginning to spread behind a dark bank of clouds. But my mind clung to my wife's image, imagining it with an uncanny acuteness. I heard her answering me, saw her smile, her frank and encouraging look. Real or not, her look was then*

more luminous than the sun which was beginning to rise.

A thought transfixed me: for the first time in my life I saw the truth as it is set into song by so many poets, proclaimed as the final wisdom by so many thinkers. The truth—that love is the ultimate and the highest goal to which man can aspire. Then I grasped the meaning of the greatest secret that human poetry and human thought and belief have to impart: The salvation of man is through love and in love. I understood how a man who has nothing left in this world still may know bliss, be it only for a brief moment, in the contemplation of his beloved. In a position of utter desolation, when man cannot express himself in positive action, when his only achievement may consist in enduring his sufferings in the right way—an honorable way—in such a position man can, through loving contemplation of the image he carries of his beloved, achieve fulfillment. For the first time in my life I was able to understand the meaning of the words, "The angels are lost in perpetual contemplation of an infinite glory."

Monks, nuns, and laypeople in the Buddhist world can take the vow of the *bodhisattva*, an idea most heavily emphasized in the Tibetan traditions. The vow is a promise to delay the attainment of their spiritual liberation, *nirvana*, for countless rebirths until all beings, human and animal, have themselves been freed from suffering by attaining *nirvana*. Whether we take this vow literally or symbolically, and whether we find its similar expression in Hindu, Muslim, Jewish, or Christian vocabularies, it reorients our position in the world—service becomes the pivot of existential meaning. As a counterpoint to the impossibility of satisfying our insatiable hungers, it's a refreshing alternative.

According to the mystics, the pursuit of our personal desires is insufficient for happiness. Frankl, Keller, and many others have said that true fulfillment in living comes from love and fidelity to a worthy purpose. Whether it's the love of a child or a spouse, or a search for the divine, or devotion to a political cause, that purpose holds more promise for real happiness than the satisfaction of our personal wants and needs.

The foundations for fulfillment, however, include having our basic physical and emotional needs met, a point made by Abraham Maslow in his well-known hierarchy of needs. Though insufficient alone for happiness, fulfilling our bodily needs is essential. Studies have shown that while earning an above-average income offers no extra measure of happiness, poverty can contribute greatly to our unhappiness and can shorten life. Certainly, financial security can contribute to peace of mind. But the theme repeats itself in spiritual traditions throughout the world: our happiness comes from contributing to others. The fundamentals of the American Dream can meet our basic physical needs without which happiness can be elusive. But the excesses of that Dream, and all our acquisitions and sensory enchantments, leave us satiated for only a fleeting moment. Redefining our lives and our identities by a worthy purpose is a surgical bypass of insatiability, helping us escape the Sisyphean task of forever trying to satisfy the implacable urge for more.

In *Man and Superman*, the ever-unabashed George Bernard Shaw wrote:

This is the true joy in life—the being used for a purpose recognized by yourself as a mighty one; the being thoroughly worn out before you are thrown on the scrap heap; the being a force of Nature instead of a feverish little clod of ailments and grievances complaining that the world will not devote itself to making you happy.

When our lives become a dedication to the welfare of others, the very ground of being changes. The reason for being alive is transformed. A rousing morning routine might be to look in the mirror before shaving or applying makeup and ask, "Am I being a feverish little clod of ailments and grievances complaining that the world will not devote itself to making me happy?"

As a psychologist at the University of Chicago, Mihaly Csikszentmihalyi (*pronounced cheek-sent-me-high*) conducted research on what constitutes a happy, fulfilled life. He and his team gave pagers to their subjects, then contacted them at random times throughout the week. They instructed the subjects to record both their activities at the moment and how happy they felt. After analyzing over a hundred thousand such data points, the team got unexpected results. In his book, *Flow: The Psychology of Optimal Experience*, Csikszentmihalyi concluded that happiness isn't derived from unlimited access to pleasure. He wrote that our happiest moments are not the leisurely, relaxing times we usually associate with happiness, and instead, they come when we are fully engaged in "voluntary efforts to accomplish something difficult and worthwhile." In other words, when we are called upon to be our best, to be creative and committed in a meaningful task, we are happiest. Csikszentmihalyi goes on to suggest that the closest we can come to anything we define as happiness is "a sense of *participation* in determining the content of life."

If you ask sick patients why they want to be healthy, they give you strange looks at first. Then, the usual answer is something like, "I just want to feel good." But if you keep probing, their comments usually point to the need for some sense of meaning and purpose. As they reflect further, it dawns on them that they want health for the freedom to contribute to the community, the world, or their children and grandchildren. They want to see their progeny turning into productive, caring citizens who will heal and strengthen the world. They want to be alive and healthy to love their grandchildren and to see them graduate, or to help their communities or the country.

We could also ask why Bill Gates, George Soros, Warren Buffett, and other wealthy people keep working. Do they need more money for a truly comfortable retirement? Then we have ripened, wrinkled elders who keep working though they have enough money for several lifetimes of leisure. Clearly, they're living with purpose. They understand that playing endless golf, traveling for months, or lying on a beach for weeks are not tickets to true fulfillment. Instead, they intuitively know that a robust engagement with life happens at the productive interface between their talents and, as Frederick Buechner says, the deep hunger of the world. They can have or do virtually anything they want, but they choose to keep working in pursuit of a different calling. This sort of satisfaction is firewood for the soul, giving it energy for healing and integration. If our entertainments are ripples on the ocean surface, meaning and purpose are the deep swelling currents below.

To live with meaning and purpose is to generate energy, and the resulting vitality then contributes to a healthier life. As Frankl, Keller, Shaw, saints, and mystics throughout the centuries have said, a life with clear, conscious meaning puts us in accord with the design of the cosmos. That meaning would ideally be a dedication to a cause or purpose greater than oneself. In a similar vein, the Dalai Lama said, "Our prime purpose in this life is to help others."

Purpose as context

Purpose and meaning point to a different texture of happiness. While pictures of children with beaming faces might come to mind as symbols of happiness, there's also another sensibility—quieter and subtler—that comes from the stillness of knowing one's purpose for being alive. That becomes the backdrop for the dancing bears of life's challenges: a sense of existential wellness that is the background for everything we do. Just as an autumn sun casts a glow of gold on an entire hillside, a context of meaning gives color to the whole of our lives.

One advantage of this perspective is that our happiness is then no longer defined by the mood du jour. Referring back to the discussion on states and stages, an emotion is a state, while living on purpose can be a stage. So a momentary state of frustration or discouragement shrinks in size when put in the context of a meaningful purpose. Purpose waits steady in the background like a watchful parent, while our emotions run about like kids on the playground.

This difference is easily illustrated in sports. When an athlete's lungs are bursting and legs are on fire, she could be having a very good time, according to Csikszentmihalyi's definition. The reason may be that the finish line is a few feet away or that she just scored a goal. In that case, the athlete wouldn't trade the pain for anything. But if we thought of bursting lungs and burning legs out of context, we'd think, how awful. It's the meaning, not the sensation, which determines whether we are thrilling or suffering.

In the summer of 2001, my son and I went on a guided expedition to the 19,343-foot summit of Mt. Kilimanjaro in Tanzania. I thought it would serve as a modern rite of passage for him around his sixteenth birthday, and a celebration of my fiftieth. After several days of a slow ascent to the camp at 15,000 feet, and after just a few hours of sleep on the third night, we started off in the sub-freezing, star-filled night at about one in the morning. At those altitudes, we could creep along for only a few minutes at a petty pace without getting breathless. For our local guides in their ragged sneakers, though, it was another casual walk.

We reached the summit, Uhuru Peak, at about nine in the morning, then walked back down to the camp at 12,000 feet by evening. We had hiked eighteen straight hours, mostly in thin air. I hadn't slept the night before because of the altitude's effects, so I'd been awake for thirty-six hours, hiking for twenty-six. I didn't know such exhaustion was humanly possible. But with my legs of lead, my impossible fatigue, and my aching body caked in grime and sunscreen, I was ecstatic. The meaning of the sensations was granted by context. I was elated at having made it to the top and at having seen my son grinning proudly on the summit with the immense African cloudscape below us. On the descent, he was so exhausted that whenever we stopped for a break, he would fall asleep sitting up, then go into hallucinatory dream states in a few seconds. Yet the climb was one of the high points of his life. A sensation is one thing, its meaning another.

Self-care and caring for others

If we are each sewn into the cloth of the world, into the fabric of the Whole, then caring for our own health is ultimately a contribution to others. Self-care is not only about our own bodies. To take good care of our souls and bodies is to take care of the world's true wealth. In *The Life We Are Given*, Michael Murphy and George Leonard addressed this point by writing, "In terms of social responsibility, the pursuit of health is a *moral* act." They were alluding to this bond with each other, a bond that is not only metaphysical but practical too, as we'll see later. Health *for* a purpose starts with seeing that our skin is more than wrapping for the package and remembering that we exist always within layer after layer of context.

Contrary to the street view of things, our health is not restricted to what's under the inside surface of our skin. To the mystic's eye, the body's interior is only one face of the universe. Since all the elements of the human body, such as carbon, hydrogen, and oxygen, are made from the ashes of big fireballs that erupted billions of years ago, we are all cut from the same cosmic cloth. If we remember that our own health, in the end, is inseparable from that of others, then it might help us stop sacrificing our health at the altar of altruism. On a flight, we're instructed to put an oxygen mask on our children only after we've put one on ourselves. We're not much help to the child when passed out on the floor. Altruism demands that we ourselves be in good enough shape to do the necessary work. It's not selfishness. Taking care of ourselves first is essential.

A useful exercise for understanding this better is to imagine how much you'll be missed once you're gone. You'll leave behind big empty spaces of longing after your death, waves of sadness that will fade slowly and become small but constant ripples like those at the lakeshore. Some of you may be thinking you shouldn't flatter yourself, but with few exceptions, we are loved. Unfortunately, the unbridled, earnest expressions of caring by your friends and loved ones usually come only in eulogy at your memorial service. Nevertheless, you are admired, appreciated, and loved now. It's not egotistical to think this, but honest. Don't those of us with deceased parents wish they were still alive, able see our children growing and thriving? I occasionally imagine my parents coming back to life, mouths agape, elated, on seeing my children as the flourishing adults they are today. For myself, of course, I miss them both—Dad since 1982, Mom since 1999. I know I'll always miss them. Like all the dead, they didn't anticipate that they were so loved that we'd be missing them for decades.

Staying robust and staying healthy—socially, financially, biologically, spiritually, psychologically—is more than your personal business. With the state of your health, you are affecting the world, if only one little corner of it. The opportunity in being healthy and full of beans is to ride the waves of human purpose, to do the tasks of the world, to weave together the fragmented pieces of humankind.

Your health is not just about prevention and the avoidance of disease, nor is it just about the satisfaction of daily concerns; rather, it is a contribution to the whole because each of us is inescapably a part of the Whole. To know and to admit that you are loved is a great gift to give your friends and family. Paradoxically, it's the absence of this knowledge that lies at the root of conceit. If you continue to abuse your health and lead yourself early into the grave, that's insensitive to those who love you. Giving nourishes both the giver and the receiver.

Designed to care

Mystics tell us that the energies of the world push for unification between people through the act of caring. It's ironic, then, that seemingly isolated individuals are not really separate in the first place. We are, in the final sense, not alone and never alone. The acts of giving and receiving make more tangible what we could call an *already-connectedness*: we are already connected to people and things, whether we feel it or not, no matter how lonely we may feel. When we breathe in, we take in one small part of an entire universe. That's not a metaphor but a literal, measurable truth. When we create a sense of communion by giving and receiving, by contributing to the world, we simply reposition ourselves in alignment with how things are already established. We know from our social norms that contributing to others is its own reward. Our designated heroes, those who evoke our most fervent admiration, are usually those who make sacrifices for another or for the common good.

This takes us back to the idea of allurement, which includes, among many things, the way people gravitate toward each other. Imagine a world in which no one wanted to live or work with others. It evokes the question of why we want to belong to a community in the first place. The innate desire for marriage, whether among the straight or gay, the built-in desire for children, for bonding with like-minded people, is the world's charisma at play. Martin Buber wrote:

> *Every true deed is a loving deed. All true deeds arise from contact with a beloved thing and flow into the universe. Any true deed brings, out of lived unity, unity into the world. Unity is not a property of the world, but its task. To form unity out of the world is our never-ending work.*

This echoes the writings of Sri Aurobindo and Teilhard de Chardin, who wrote that the drive toward wholeness is the task of a conscious, intelligent universe. Brian Swimme, as we have seen, calls it allurement. Stanislav Grof writes of the Cosmic Game. Ken Wilber and Andrew Cohen speak of the evolutionary impulse. Mystics from cultures around the globe have said this in a thousand ways: the ground of being is not neutral but loving, asking for union between people. If we look under the stones of apathy or antagonism, we will find the authentic self as a thing of love and beauty. Whether we chat and mingle with friends, melt into sexual bliss with a lover, or volunteer at a hospital, we engage in what Buber calls the task of the world, the task of creating unity, a task that's in the design of the cosmos. While we might think of such urges as only personally ours, and while that's true in one sense, they're enfolded within progressively bigger shells of meaning like Russian nesting dolls. Our personal desires are the smallest doll.

Some would argue that the evidence points overwhelmingly to the selfishness and violence in human nature. War, crime, wealth disparities, racial prejudice, and callousness toward the environment all point to our animalistic nature. Newspapers are filled with stories of decadence, depravity, terrorism, genocide, the intransigence in the Middle East, the intractability of global poverty. The world is on fire, and this, they say, demonstrates the idiocy of human nature with its primordial egocentrism, *Lord of the Flies* writ large. This view, supported by centuries of anecdotal evidence, is also supported by Freudian theory which sees human nature as being driven by the *id*—that uncivilized, self-centered, primitive part of ourselves. This *id* must be controlled by the *superego*, which is the voice of civility and moral sensibilities. Without the superego, the uncivilized self throws itself onto the world without an ethical compass.

My patient Eric questions the shape of existential design. Both his parents were crazy and abusive, he said. His father would often leave his wife and children to ride the rails as a hobo for weeks on end. One day, he told the eight-year-old Eric of his intentions to eventually kill himself, and a few years later, made good on the promise. Shortly thereafter, Eric's mother also committed suicide. His sister took her life when she was thirty-two. At nineteen, Eric married a seventeen-year-old with severe psychiatric disorders who later would be institutionalized for most of her life. When she wasn't in the hospital, she would hit and scream at their children, and once even tried to drown two of them. As the children grew older, one jumped off a five-story building in a suicide attempt, though she survived to live with a damaged brain and a broken body.

Today, Eric is on many medications for diabetes, congestive heart failure, polymyalgia rheumatica, kidney disease, and five other medical conditions. His aging body hurts terribly, and he is convinced that his physical ailments are trumpets of the emotional suffering he has endured. To use his words, the agonies of his life were more than any single human being should have to bear. And at one point, he shook his head to say, "If something created the universe, he/she/it is a lunatic." That reminds me of listening to Elie Wiesel speak in Washington, D.C. many years ago. Toward the end of his talk, he said that the Holocaust shook his faith in God, and since then, he hasn't been able to reconcile the horrors perpetrated during that time with the idea of a benevolent God.

The question of evil has plagued theologians and philosophers for centuries, a question for which a tightly packaged answer is not on the horizon of human inquiry and certainly not in this book. But even in the face of horrors such as the genocides of the Holocaust, Rwanda, and Pol Pot's Cambodia, there are signs of benevolence in the design of things.

The sorry state of human affairs is not proof of an essential callousness in human nature, no more than our personal transgressions are the final arbiter of whether we're good or bad at heart. True, the shadows of human nature can create untold mayhem, and the malevolence of tyrants can't be explained away simplistically as neurosis or compensation for an unhappy childhood. While those who harm others have often been victims of childhood abuse themselves, the unspeakable evil of many dictators begs for a heftier philosophical explanation, one delving into highly complex questions of good and evil. But the possibility that we're good at heart—in essence, and underneath all our defenses, denials, and social camouflage—isn't negated by the reality that we have evil of colossal proportions in the world, evidenced by individuals such as Pol Pot, Stalin, and Hitler. At the very least, we have statistical muscle to support the essential goodness of humankind: for every criminal act in the world, there are a million acts of civility at the supermarket, in the office, on the sidewalks.

When Buber wrote, "Every true deed is a loving deed," he put forth not just a psychological notion but the philosophical view that the design of human nature was embedded in the blueprint of the cosmos. He points to the essential goodness within, stating that when we act in a loving way, we are aligned with our true nature. Conversely, when we are selfish, resentful, or violent, we are, ultimately, inauthentic. The book *A Course in Miracles* conveys the same idea: "Every loving thought is true, and everything else is an appeal for help and healing no matter what form it takes." *A Course* states that peeling off the defenses, masks, and compensations from the surfaces of human nature will reveal a loving self. It is fear, arising out of our estrangement from the authentic self, that leads to self-aggrandizement, cruelty, and heartlessness. Once we assuage this fear, we will discover the caring self inside. If we can remember that the neuroses, transgressions, and insensitivities of others are mirages, the sting of their words will either decrease or disappear.

I had the "Every loving thought" quote taped on my refrigerator for years. As I looked at the challenges in my personal and professional relationships through the lens of this idea, it helped me remain less convinced when people tried their best to persuade me of their belligerence or insensitivity. If we consciously choose to view people as essentially benevolent, we're less likely to be fooled by their façade of bullying, bitterness, or boasting. If we assume that fear conceals goodness even as it knocks all the china off the shelf, we will inhabit a different world, one populated with people who are willing to love at the slightest nudge. By assuming the stance that people are essentially loving, although some of them happen not to have been so informed, we can transform relationships. Later, we'll see how Karen, whom we've already met, transformed her relationships with her brothers using this idea.

Giving

Many people think of our capacity to give as a fixed quantity, like water in a bucket. Once we've given away all our water, our bucket's empty and we're depleted.

That's a myth. There's a difference between the art of giving and the threads of dissonance we easily weave into that art. What causes fatigue is not the giving, but dissonance. Whether in professional or personal relationships, this comes in many forms. It comes about when we dislike anything, to any degree, in ourselves or in the other.

We might doubt our competence. We might feel that the caring transaction is unfair—I'm giving more than I'm getting. We might be frustrated that the recipients of our help are hell-bent on destroying themselves in spite of our best efforts and highest intentions. We might be resentful that they repeatedly reject our attempts to help. We might be judgmental about their need to be rescued from the consequences of their irresponsible behavior. We might be bored with the routine after twenty or thirty years. In short, it's this hand-wringing, brow-knitting, and hair-tearing that depletes us, not the giving itself, nor the behavior of others.

Fatigue from giving also often comes from neglecting our own needs for rest, relaxation, exercise, and nourishment for both the body and soul. Guilt often drives the fixation on giving until depleted, as we may have been taught early in our lives that caring for our own needs is selfish. In that scenario, it's either/or: either they or I will thrive, but not both. If one wins, the other suffers. Today, we can easily see the confusion behind that belief. Self-neglect, and even self-abuse masquerading as largesse, are as different from caring as masochism is different from the enjoyment of sports.

So it's the angst and drama, along with self-neglect, that deplete energy. But unadulterated giving does not. If we give freely and authentically, we can even create more energy, as we've seen. Pearl Bailey captured this idea when she wrote:

> *I see their souls*
> *and I hold them in my hands,*
> *and because I love them,*
> *they weigh nothing.*

If she loves them, they weigh nothing. The giving is not transactional. I take this as more than a reflection on the lovability of our friends; rather, a suggestion that when feeling wholly resonant and unfettered in our giving, we ourselves also weigh nothing in the transparency of a calm heart. When giving is free of drama, it's effortless, like water flowing serenely around stones. At those times, both the giver and receiver weigh nothing.

But many people are in circumstances that would run roughshod over the most thoughtfully cultivated attitudes. Caring nonstop for a dying spouse for months on end, working a frenzied nightshift in the emergency room, or sleeping minimally while working in a refugee camp—all demand an imposing amount of stamina. But examining and working through our internal dissonance—the guilt, compulsions, anxieties, and so on—will help keep our coffers of energy better stocked in most circumstances.

Beyond the psychological view of this idea, we also have the philosophical view. Perhaps the act of giving is both socially valued and inherently gratifying because, as Buber said, it's the task of the universe. In other words, contributing to others may be part of the design of it all. A friend or patient looking at you with grateful eyes, a child thrilled by your gift, or a friend hugging and squeezing you in appreciation are infusions of perfume into our souls which we could explain in purely personal, psychological terms. But many mystics and philosophers have suggested that it's more than personal, that it instead is designed into the architecture of the cosmos. When we give, we get energy back because we're better aligned with the metaphysical blueprints. With that in mind, many have said that giving is receiving. St. Francis, for one, said so: "It is in giving that we receive."

In this view, giving sustains the giver because it's part of the plan. Since we have already looked at health as not just the absence of disease, nor just vibrancy in mind and body, but as part of a transformative journey, then *giving is a component of health*. This applies to giving in all its forms. It is life, and therefore health, flourishing as it recreates itself.

Over the years, I've learned that any fatigue I feel from my work comes not from giving, but from my doubts and anxieties. If I'm distracted, uncertain, judgmental, or frustrated, then tiredness comes quickly like a pouncing cat. If, on the other hand, I feel fully engaged and confident, I'm spirited all day. In fact, I can become more energetic as the day goes on. In the long run, the gratification of having helped many people, in spite of my failures to help many others, is itself a priceless source of energy.

This became clear to me during a flight out of a snowy Cincinnati many years ago. Because the wing flaps froze into place minutes after takeoff, the jet had to return to the airport for an emergency landing. Because the pilot was unable to control the flaps, he was unable to control the speed. So we were to risk a high-speed landing back at the airport. As the plane descended too rapidly toward the runway, the flight attendants told us to cross our hands on the seat in front of us, then to put our foreheads on them. We were as silent as ice. You could feel the fear in the cabin. As we approached the runway, we could see fire trucks and ambulances lined up, waiting for us. While I sat with my forehead pressed against the seat in front of me, I thought about my possible death. I felt a wave of sadness that I might not see my family and loved ones again, but as I thought of how I'd done the best I could for them and for the people I'd helped through my work, I felt a soft wave of peacefulness come through my body. I was ready. Since I had a hefty life insurance policy, I also noted the irony of being worth more dead than alive. We banged onto that runway far too hard and the engines roared far too long, but we were safe. The discovery that I felt existentially complete was liberating.

Receiving

Ironically, many of us find it harder to receive than to give. The merits of receiving a gift graciously are well understood, but still, we're often awkward recipients. Perhaps that comes from thinking we're undeserving, or from feeling embarrassed by the benevolence of others, or from many other reasons. We might have learned as children to sacrifice our own needs in order to ward off accusations of being selfish. On the other hand, we might be too enamored with feeling magnanimous as the giver. And being the receiver might have us feeling weak, needy, or inferior. But there is an intriguing aspect to giving and receiving that often goes unnoticed. To illustrate, I'll highlight one part of *The Man of La Mancha*, the musical based on *Don Quixote* by Miguel Cervantes.

On his journey to vanquish the forces of evil and become a knight, the grandiose, hyperbolic Don Quixote and his sidekick, Sancho Panza, stay at an inn where he meets the innkeeper, some rowdy guests, and the miserable maid and harlot, Aldonzo. Bitter, foul-mouthed, and unkempt, she is angry at her lowly life and over the indignities she suffers at the hands of men. But Don Quixote, with his delusional exuberance, sees her as the Princess Dulcinea— an elegant and beautiful apparition who is part of his heroic quest. This is destiny, he thinks, since every knight on a sacred quest must have a princess at his side. He pours on the praise for her beauty and royal lineage, but to no avail—she is uninterested. In fact, she finds his delusions repellent. Since Aldonzo is clearly a bitter and wretched woman, Don Quixote's affections seem grossly misplaced.

As the story unfolds, Don Quixote continues with his quest that is marked by one defeat after another. After all his brawls and scuffles, he meets Dulcinea again toward the end. But by now, she has been transformed into the dignified, beautiful woman that he had always imagined her to be. We see that his love, his impossibly delightful affirmation of her worth, helped her discover her own elegance and grace. Don Quixote's convictions were catalysts for the change, and she changed only after she welcomed his gifts. The Don himself was ecstatic, though he'd never expected anything less. What happened is described by a quote from James Elkins, who wrote:

> *Ultimately, seeing alters the thing that is seen and transforms the seer. Seeing is a metamorphosis, not a mechanism.*

We could also say that caring alters the person cared for and transforms the giver, that caring is a metamorphosis, not a mechanism. While we'd normally think of vision as a way of getting information, and of giving as an act symbolized by the transference of water from one bucket to another, the quote from Elkins and the story of Dulcinea tell us otherwise: perception, and caring, have transforming effects. Giving and receiving are catalysts for change. They signify the creative, generative power of love.

So this is what we do with our loved ones, especially our children, who know themselves and become themselves through our love. When we believe in others and love them, they are made whole. With this in mind, the bucket-of-water model—the transactional view of giving—seems mechanistic. That model involves two buckets, whereas mystics say that the giver and receiver are merely different sides of the same coin, profoundly related to each other. Through giving and receiving, they come to know each other more fully, to express their true nature, to be more alive because they are more real. Giving and receiving create knowledge, not as data, but as the wisdom that aligns us with the architecture of the cosmos.

In the Hindu traditions, especially those related to what's known as Advaita Vedanta, a core belief is that there is only one consciousness, and we are each an integral part of it. The idea was echoed in Carl Jung's idea of the collective unconscious, an ocean of consciousness to which our individual minds are connected as rivers and streams.

To return to the idea that "caring is metamorphosis," a good example is found in child development. Infants who are loved and nurtured develop their neurological and behavioral potential, but feral, isolated, or unloved children do not. The parts of the brain used in learning language, abstractions, and relationship skills develop only when the child is loved, stimulated, and nurtured. After a narrow window of time in their early years, the chances of later developing those brain functions are very low. They need love to flourish.

Of course, adults too need love to flourish. My patient Alan was a senior executive who spent weeks in intensive care with a burst aneurysm in his brain. The bleeding had been brought under control, but there was a risk it might worsen. And if it got worse, he would die. For many weeks, he teetered on the thin edge between life and death. His friends and family were devastated, his wife frantic.

During his hospitalization, friends and family sent Alan a flood of good wishes through a free website called CaringBridge. The site is designed for communication with those stricken by an illness and allows a friend or family member to post updates on the patient's progress. These can be read by everyone interested, an arrangement that saves the trouble of endless phone calls and email updates from those already under enough stress. In Alan's situation, friends, coworkers, and relatives by the dozen sent messages of love and encouragement. His wife would then print them and read them aloud to him whenever he was conscious.

After the crisis, Alan's life was transformed. He worked less, ate better, exercised and relaxed more. His priorities were completely upended. He resolved to work forty hours a week, not sixty. He dropped his cigarettes like a hot stone. He spent more time with his family. After being millimeters from death, he recognized what was truly important to him: his family. Of the many lessons he learned from this crisis, Alan was especially moved by the outpouring of concern and well wishes. He was stunned by the more than 2,300 messages of love and caring he received through the website. As a result, he changed his priorities, placing love and family before work. After the crisis was over, he said that he had no doubts that the love he felt through the messages helped with his recovery. Like Dulcinea, he was made whole by the love and compassion sent his way.

Those lucky enough to have a strong social network are usually flooded with cards, calls, and flowers while hospitalized. After the crisis, they invariably say how surprised and moved they were by the show of concern, almost disbelieving how blind they'd been to their importance to others. They often say that this love and appreciation was essential for their recovery. Being a willing recipient helped them heal.

Before moving on, we have more on the subject of giving and receiving worth considering.

The effect on the giver

Another idea that rarely gets much attention is the effect that receiving has on the giver. When we receive, the fidgeting, awkward focus on ourselves leads us to forget that the giver is enriched by the act of giving. When the role is reversed and we're in the role of the giver, we might feel queasy, or even offended, when someone rejects our gifts out of politeness. But what's missing there is the awareness that we feel ennobled by our own generosity.

We get a hint of this from how we responded when, in his inaugural address, John F. Kennedy Jr. told the nation, "Ask not what your country can do for you, but what you can do for your country." We weren't offended; we were inspired. His meta-message was that we could be trusted for our nobler instincts, and this reinforced our moral stature by implying that Americans can rise above petulant individualism. We approved of him because he trusted our largesse. The call to a spirit of service didn't have us dig in with the heels of narcissism, but on the contrary, had us more inclined to be altruistic.

Living in commitment and with purpose

Living with purpose helps sustain health. With a commitment to something greater than oneself, the experience of being alive is given richer meaning. Commitment infuses the body with energy. The urge to contribute is reflected in the words of Rilke when he wrote, "The god wants to know himself in you." If each of us is an aperture through which the universe is trying to know itself, then living with purpose corresponds with the design of the world. This may not come naturally to us, but that doesn't invalidate the idea that we may be designed to contribute. Maturing into an ethos of generosity and contribution may be one of the central tasks of our spiritual and moral development.

Meaning and purpose in my search for wholeness

Not too many years after I returned from Sri Lanka, I set up a private practice in acupuncture and settled into a relatively normal American life. It was a long way from exotic lands and the austerities of Asian monasticism.

Since my years in Sri Lanka, I've come to see much that I couldn't see then. I see now that going to a quiet monastery in another world, shaving my head and wearing simple robes and giving up all comforts, was, in the end, no less hedonistic than the way I'd conducted myself before. That may sound like stretching definitions here, but I saw that we can be spiritually narcissistic and spiritually hedonistic if the obsession is simply to give ourselves pleasure, however esoteric. A good example of this can be found in the gist of much prayer: please give me what I want. In dire times, many people will start bargaining: I'll sacrifice something but only if I get something in return. However, I don't consider that a problem. The reason is that we can't start enlightened or begin whole. If we drive head-on into spiritual work, at least we're on the right racetrack—however small our engines, however elementary our driving skills.

The problem with pleasure, even when it results from spiritual practices, is that it's smoke. It vanishes. Even if we could endlessly stimulate pleasure, physical or mental, it will eventually fade because the nervous system habituates quickly and can't sustain feeling good indefinitely. We know how a thrill made perpetual becomes boring. The tingling in our toes from getting the home or car of our dreams eventually wears off. We might continue to feel a sense of satisfaction from the home or the car, but sooner or later, we'd have to admit that the thrill is gone. Researchers have set up laboratory experiments in which the brains of rats would release dopamine, through either electrical stimulation or the administration of a drug, each time the rats pressed a lever. Dopamine is a neurochemical that produces sensations of wellbeing and is involved in the reward and punishment system in the nervous system. Its fluctuations are part of the mechanisms of addiction. The rats became so obsessed with the pleasure, often ignoring food and rest, that in the end, trying to pleasure themselves in this way, they became completely exhausted. Some even died of starvation because they didn't bother to eat.

They killed themselves trying to feel good.

This is where the elegance of Buddhist principles comes in. Stated in contemporary and highly simplified terms, one of the principles is that it's awfully hard to be happy all the time. Sure, we'll have good moments, plenty of them, but once they're gone, they're gone like yesterday's sunshine. All those moments of ecstasy—the triumphs, the euphoric sex, the island vacations, the first month of retirement, the promotions, the wedding day—they're done, gone, defunct. This, by the way, is not cynicism or pessimism. If you warn your toddler not to run out in front of a moving truck, that doesn't make you a pessimist. Nor does this principle have anything to do with resignation or passivity. It's simply sidestepping the trap of living in the circularity of dissatisfaction.

We've heard much of positivity and affirmations lately, and I think they're terrific. But taken to an extreme, they can lead to a fear of admitting to hard truths. So the idea that pleasure is ephemeral, like smoke, is a precursor to good news. It may be one of the secrets behind the high-wattage smiles of the monks at Kanduboda—they understood how to detour around the dead-end routes. They were released.

Over the years, it started to get clearer to me. The race is not to the swift. In our inner worlds, there is no race.

I've experienced big wins, heavy losses, great jobs, humiliations, a rewarding professional practice. But a relentless thirst remained, one that my time in Sri Lanka was to have satisfied. Over the years, a theme emerged, one that seemed a natural complement to the insatiability of this existential thirst. It was encapsulated in the quote from Helen Keller earlier in this chapter, and in others such as this from de Chardin:

The most satisfying thing in life is to have been able to give
a large part of one's self to others.

Living with a meaningful purpose, perhaps even one you would die for, paves the potholes of daily living. In my earlier years, I often thought about the altruism of people such as Florence Nightingale, Albert Schweitzer, the Dalai Lama, Harriet Tubman, and Nelson Mandela. Then there were those we read about in the newspapers, including elementary school children, passionate in their dedication to the poor and the sick. I, on the other hand, was too absorbed in myself to have that kind of character; I decided I wasn't designed with such a heroic outlook on social concerns.

The break came when I realized it wasn't necessarily a matter of character. I began to see that living with purpose could be a choice, independent of character or inclination, and that a wholly legitimate way of being myself could be formed by the simple act of declaration.

The fresh new idea for me was that the act of speaking brings forth worlds. If I say my life is a dedication to the health and wellbeing of humankind, then it's so just because I said so. If I promise to meet you for lunch on Tuesday, that promise is a type of truth. Not all things work that way—the earth revolves around the sun whether we say it does or not—but some things do.

Simply declaring the intention to be an advocate of the world is like creating a sculpture. It now exists because we made it. The good news is that we don't need a ready-made selflessness, an intrinsic altruism, or a genetic proclivity to lead a solicitous life. I had none of that. I had overdosed on anxiety about hell and bore the footprints of boot-camp style castigations on my psyche. My focus was emotional survival. The resulting need to fill the hungers of body and soul, my unhappiness during my earlier years, were not exactly precursors to a life of purpose.

Instead, by simply choosing to reposition myself in my world toward service, I've found much gratification in the meaning it provides. It's about being embedded in the web of human consequence, of contributing one small bit to the world's work, of standing on the planet in a posture of support.

It's not a feeling, but a still, quiet place that becomes a context for living—which, incidentally, improves the likelihood of enjoying its byproducts such as sensations of joy and pleasure. Byproduct is the key word here. If we live on purpose, our mood at any given moment becomes less of a concern.

None of this disavows the primitive human needs that are my inheritance. Too many of our most astute observers of the human condition, including Stanislav Grof, Ken Wilber, Fritz Perls, and Carl Jung, have been telling us we can't be whole without integrating the primitive, animal self into a more sophisticated form of selfhood.

Raw, primal instinct, instead of being a demon to conquer, can be recruited and redirected toward the greater good. This channeling of energy can enliven our animal soul, creating even more energy for change. It's crucial to know this, as we can't will away the animal self or the obsession with *me* by shoving them into a cage of suppression and hoping they'll die of starvation. That would be a fundamentalist approach—the school of *just say no*—which can lead to a bloating of passions, and in the worst case, to violence and mayhem.

Instead, the natural, inevitable concern for *I, me, mine* can be redirected and integrated into our travels toward the higher good. I've come to see that living with purpose circumvents the insatiability of my appetites. The strategy is no longer to eat as much as I can in the hopes of fulfilling those hungers.

I'll conclude with more from Buber:

Free is the man that wills without caprice. He believes in the actual, which is to say: he believes in the real association of the real duality, I and You. He believes in destiny and also that it needs him. It does not lead him, it waits for him. He must proceed toward it without knowing where it waits for him. He must go forth with his whole being: that he knows. It will not turn out the way his resolve intended it; but what he wants to come will come only if he resolves to do that which he can will. He must sacrifice his little will, which is unfree and ruled by things and drives, for his great will that moves away from being determined to find destiny. Now he no longer interferes, nor does he merely allow things to happen. He listens to what grows, to the way of Being in the world, not in order to be carried along by it but rather in order to actualize it in the manner in which it, needing him, wants to be actualized by him—with human spirit and human deed, with human life and human death. He believes, I said; but this implies: he encounters.

What a surprising thought: the possibility that we are needed by destiny, the great will, to do its work.

To exist is to be related—however invisible, elusive, or indirect the connection—to everyone else. However isolated we may feel, we're snug with the world. Even when alone and lonely in a cold apartment on a winter night, we live in this unison, surrounded by the scent of devotion, verve, and the promise of exhilaration. In a similar way, health is more than a condition of the internal physical landscape planted with glands, hormones, and enzymes. It reveals itself at the interface between our individual selves and the World, the omniverse. The two-way road of giving and receiving broadens that interface, and accordingly, helps us become healthier. This intimacy is a fluid, dynamic border that connects us to the world. When Buber writes of sacrificing the little will for the great will which needs us to do its work, he points to a context of meaning surrounding us: we're here for a purpose, and that purpose is grander than our own individual designs for our lives. Health, as an alignment with our full potentiality, is served well by living on purpose in a world of deep meaning. James Joyce wrote:

Welcome, O life! I go to encounter for the millionth time
the reality of experience and to forge in the smithy of my soul
the uncreated conscience of my race.

Chapter Seven

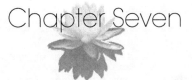

Nourish: The Breath of Flowers

Whole, natural foods are sculptures, created not by the earth but by the artistry of its wisdom. Growing out of soil with a heritage of fourteen billion years, they're molded by nature's creativity in a fairly good approximation of something being created out of nothing. Since to the best of our knowledge nothing existed before the Big Bang, everything that exists has ultimately been created out of nothing. But what's been sculpted is more than just beautiful art. It's intelligence embodied, smarts alive. Broccoli, tomato, cantaloupe, coconut, the flesh of animals, and all whole foods are packed with information and possibility compatible with the genetic software of the human body.

An orange, for example, has over three hundred nutrients to which our cells give full diplomatic recognition. Our cells understand the software program called orange, but not the one called potato chip. When we eat whole foods, we absorb the wisdom of the universe that propels the evolution of the human body. Fresh, whole, natural foods deepen our intimacy with the world. They animate us. While all this sounds like metaphor for hard truths, Plato would have insisted on the reverse, saying that what's visible is the metaphor.

Similar to what I've done in previous chapters when discussing the body and its symptoms, I will emphasize not the specifics of nutrition, but its essence. Thousands of books on nutrition and a surfeit of theories are available today, and it's not the purview of this book to explore them. I will instead look at two ideas: the soul and essence of nourishment and exercise, and the challenges of implementing the knowledge we already have.

I chose this approach because in my years of practice, I have yet to meet an adult who didn't already know that vegetables are good for you and cookies are not. On the scale of public health policy, we certainly need much more education on nutrition. But a good many of us don't need to learn how to drive the car of nutrition. We simply need to find the motivation to go from neutral into first gear. To a large extent, we already know what makes for a healthy diet. But we're often stuck in the quicksand of habit, comfortably in bed with a culture of indulgence, mesmerized by the allure of cake and cola, chip and pretzel, and all manner of smartly engineered, ingeniously marketed foods.

Just as we inquired into the intelligence hidden inside the symptom, we can inquire into the essence of good nutrition and search for the truths hidden behind the skin of potatoes and peaches. Just as we've considered the body, its symptoms, our thoughts and feelings as ripples on an ocean of mysteries, we can view whole foods in the same way and look under the surface for their essential core.

Nutrition as a celebrity

After decades of being ignored, nutrition is finally getting the attention it deserves. In the 1970s, the quiet voices of nutrition advocates were muffled by the louder yawns of most of the scientific community. Most scientists and clinicians back then believed nutrition had little relevance to disease. In all fairness, that period of time came just after the era of magazine ads in which doctors, dentists, babies, and Santa Claus endorsed cigarettes. A gallon of gasoline cost thirty-three cents, car radios were all static, my health insurance cost thirty-five dollars a month, and I believe my tuition at James Madison was about three hundred dollars a semester.

Today, nutrition is not only big news; it's a star. Spas, resorts, hotels, and cruise ships now cater to the nutritional concerns of their customers. A few school systems in the country are starting to provide healthier lunches for our children. In the 1970s, *Prevention* was one of the few nutrition magazines available. Today, the landscape is unrecognizable, swarming with magazines, TV shows, infomercials, websites, professional journals, and books on nutrition bringing us a steady diet of news and the latest research on herbs, supplements, health foods, weight-loss programs, and so on.

In clinical practice, nutrition has also become more prominent. Naturopathy, for example, is a type of medicine based on a philosophy of natural healing with nutrition as one of its cornerstones, and is quickly becoming more popular. Nutritionists and dietitians have also become more numerous in recent years. Herbal medicine has become better accepted since research has shown us the life-giving potential of gingko, hawthorn, ginger, turmeric, green tea, dark chocolate, resveratrol found in red wine, and hundreds of other healing substances in roots, plants, bark, leaves, and berries. Ayurvedic medicine has long been rooted in herbalism and diet, and, through the books and lectures of Dr. Deepak Chopra, has become more familiar to the American public. Other traditional forms of healing—from Tucson to Tehran to Tibet to Taiwan to Tokyo—have extolled the power of herbs and good nutrition for over three thousand years. They continue to grow in popularity.

A small but growing number of doctors are using nutrition as a key therapeutic tool. As an example, the Institute of Functional Medicine is a nonprofit association for physicians and other professionals practicing nutrition therapy and other holistic methods of healing. With an emphasis on scientific evidence for nutrition and supplementation, the Institute supports a new, growing model of practice that highlights natural healing potential. If trends over the last thirty years are any indication, the interest in nutrition will only bloom more over the coming decades. Just a few decades ago, a membership in an organization like the Institute of Functional Medicine might have been embarrassing to a physician. Today, many professionals feel that the Institute and other such organizations represent an innovative edge of medicine.

If there's a common refrain among patients these days, it's that they don't like taking medications. The plenitude of side effects and the high costs often lead people to swallow medications with a dose of reluctance, if not distaste. Just as public demand boosted the growth of integrative medicine in the last two decades, trends suggest that it will similarly spark the continued growth of nutrition counseling, if only because it's safer. The tomato is unlikely to be recalled. Overall, the demand for natural healing methods in general has been surging steadily for three decades now and shows no sign of abating.

The essence of nutrition: to nourish

First, as we begin to explore nutrition's essence, I'll start by replacing the word nutrition with nourishment. To nourish is to help someone or something live, grow, and develop, and to become or remain healthy.

If whole foods are songs of the earth's intelligence, then ingesting them helps us tune in to that intelligence. Whole foods are an umbilical cord to possibility, to the potential tucked into the cells of the human body and into the visceral powers of the earth. The pea, carrot, asparagus, and mango all speak a language understood well by our bodies. In the way we've considered the body a concrete reflection of intangible wisdom, we can think of whole foods not as things but as forms of communication from the anima mundi, the wisdom of the world. Because they link us to the wellspring of healing, they are excellent medicine.

Of the three types of treatment methods we've examined—control, substitute, and catalyze—whole foods are catalytic. Or, more accurately, they are alchemical: the peach and tomato become you. Foods that grow out of the earth, and the animals that can grow by eating them or each other, aren't substitutes for anything. They're catalysts for our growth and transformation. In a truly alchemical way, whole foods are transformed into the human experience, and then accordingly into art, theatre, literature, religion, politics, economics, and so on. Zitkala Sa was speaking literally when she said spiritual wisdom is to be found in the sweet breathing of flowers. With a wink to this idea, Joseph Campbell once said, "A vegetarian is someone not sensitive enough to hear a carrot scream."

The growth of a small seed into a carrot or a cucumber is virtuoso performance art. First there was nearly nothing, just a genetic blueprint and a small grainy object that a bird could swallow in a quick gulp. Then there's an orange, a bean, a turnip, or a pear. The growth of a seed into a green bean is a beautifully orchestrated sign of intelligence in the universe. Whole foods are made mostly of carbon, hydrogen, and oxygen, just like our bodies. Plants breathe in air, ingest soil nutrients, produce offspring, and eliminate waste—in principle, just as human bodies do. Plants are heliotropic, following the sun in the way some people on the East Coast go to Florida every winter.

> ...the voice of the Great Spirit is heard in the twittering of birds, the rippling of mighty waters, and the sweet breathing of flowers.
>
> –Gertrude Simmons Bonnin (Zitkala Sa), Dakota Sioux

When we eat whole foods, we ingest the fertility of the universe and reinforce our primordial bond with the earth's imagination and dreams. We pay our respects to this heritage, warming to the spirit of the creative intelligence that was here long before we were born.

Whole foods are untouched, unadulterated, unprocessed foods. They come straight from nature in the form of nuts, seeds, grains, fruit, vegetables, eggs, fish, and animals. They grew into their current shape. Sometimes we find a thin line between whole and processed foods, with oils and bread being good examples. If we apply strict standards to this, bread and pasta are not whole foods, but processed ones.

Let's say that whole foods are those not coming off a factory line, those whose biochemical architecture hasn't been touched. We usually find them on the perimeter of the supermarket in the produce, meat, fish, and dairy sections.

As we saw in Chapter Three, a catalytic method elicits potential. In this sense, whole foods catalyze: they help the cell develop heft, muscle, and fitness within its walls. They help it perform its role of workhorse. They allow the communication network between the cells and between our glands and organs to work as designed. In constant negotiation, the cells talk, bargain, and trade with each other in the intercellular marketplace. This in turn leads to the market equilibrium that helps the body to grow and to repair itself. In the way the internet allows for communication in society, so the nutrients in whole foods allow for the human body's internal communication pathways to work. In order for these systems to be at their peak, we need to feed them high-quality data such as carrot or cauliflower. Carrots and cauliflower are not objects. They are information. If we ingest garbled, illogical data like potato chips or candy bars that confuse the translators in the cell, the data is not only useless to the body, but eventually harmful.

Food as a message

The idea that food is a message comes from a new direction in nutrition research. It's called nutrigenomics, which, in brief, is the study of how foods turn genes on and off. It sees food as not only fuel and building blocks for the body, but as switch operators for our genes. It explores the way food can activate or deactivate certain genes in what's known as gene expression.

As we know, genes play an important role in health and disease. Some are foundational in the onset of certain diseases like breast cancer or colon cancer, and identifying them has led science in promising new directions. But now nutrigenomics tells us that foods can awaken dormant genes and put others to sleep. As you might expect, the research shows that whole foods like broccoli and blueberries can hush the genes responsible for inflammation, weight gain, blood sugar excesses, and even the mechanisms of cancer. On the other hand, sugar, trans fats, preservatives, additives, and snack foods can activate those genes. This mechanism is similar to an internet filter for children that screens out unsavory programs and allows access only to kid-friendly ones. In this light, the role of food as an intelligent communicator with our cells is not metaphorical but literal. One of the exciting implications is that each of us has the power to influence gene expression positively through a healthy diet and lifestyle.

All this is informed by another field of study called epigenetics, in which scientists have discovered an on-off switch called an epigenome sitting atop the gene. While the genes themselves take many generations to change, epigenomes can be activated or silenced in not only a single lifetime, but in as little as a few months. What activates or silences the epigenome, and therefore the activity of the gene, is lifestyle, including exercise and diet.

One of the intriguing and reassuring implications of all this is that DNA is not destiny. This is especially noteworthy for those prone to fatalistic moods upon noting the worrisome genetic history of their families. Through an invigorating exercise program, a diet of lively, colorful, fresh foods, and a healthy soul, we can influence the orchestra of gene expression.

In this light, it should be noted that an excess of calories is overwhelming to the cells and can affect gene expression for the worse. For many years now, research has suggested that caloric restriction helps us live longer. Study after study has shown that when animals are fed a low-calorie diet, they live longer than their equals eating the usual amount of calories. While the studies have been conducted on animals only, it's considered a reasonable scientific leap to translate these effects to human physiology. Scientists are confident it's relevant to humans because the evidence is so strong in these studies on animals, from worms to mice to monkeys. It also complements the many studies showing that being obese, and even being moderately overweight, can shorten life and increase the chances of becoming sick.

It won't be surprising to learn that two key influences on the epigenomes are nutrition and exercise. Whole, nutritionally dense foods turn on the fat-burning, immune-boosting, brain-expanding, energy-stoking genes. Processed foods, which are only impostors and caricatures, activate those responsible for inflammation, oxidation, and other unhealthy conditions. Knowing how quickly gene expression can be changed, how long its effects are sustained, and how sensitive it is to lifestyle can be a great motivation to make lifestyle changes.

Here's an intriguing discovery: some studies suggest that if you eat excess calories for just one year and gain weight, you'll have increased the likelihood of a weight problem in not only your unborn children but in your unborn grandchildren. Although your genes involved in weight gain won't have changed, their epigenomes will have been activated. Over millions of years, your body has been trained to believe that a steady stream of calories is never assured, as famine often follows bounty. In its wise strategy to prepare for famine, it will store alternate sources of energy in the form of fat around the waist and hips.

Once the epigenomes responsible for this weight gain have been activated, this activation can be transmitted to your children and then again to their children. This means that if you overeat, then gain weight and lose it all in any given year, thirty years later, your adult children may be more likely to gain weight. And so will your grandchildren sixty years later. Though the genes themselves remain unchanged, the roll call for active duty was changed by diet. Stress, exercise, and the shape of your lifestyle will switch epigenomes on or off. Our relationship to future generations and the world at large is made poignant, clear, and immediate here—a good reminder of how the Iroquois believe that all our decisions and actions today should benefit the next seven generations of our children.

Broccoli, apple, kale, banana, carrot, pear, tomato, apple, mushroom, peach, pear, avocado, asparagus, lettuce, onion, blueberry, strawberry, raspberry, mango, cherry, cucumber, pepper, orange, kale, green bean, wild salmon, trout, halibut, and grass-fed organic beef, chicken, pork, and lamb... these are not foods as we have previously thought of them. We could more accurately call them intelligently programmed information systems, though you shouldn't use this term when ordering in a restaurant. Better yet, we could call them the milk of the earth and the breath of the gods. Regardless of what we call them, they're ready to tell your cancer-provoking, heart-disease-rendering, diabetes-triggering, Alzheimer's-prone genes to stand silently in the corner. Whole foods are information packets, productivity software, encoded communications, instruction manuals. They are teachers, educators, counselors, coaches, motivators, therapists. They communicate with our cells in understandable language with information packets bearing names like potassium and magnesium. They persuade the cells to perk up, to live up to their job description.

Conversely, the cells get confused by the language of sham substances like preservatives, food coloring, trans fats, partially hydrogenated oil, high fructose corn syrup, and the like. These substances are literally not food. Which means that a large portion of what the average American eats is not food.

Damaging effects of processed foods

Cakes, pies, cookies, desserts, chips, and much of what you see in the supermarket aisle are trauma to our cells. Foods wrapped in plastic, with an ingredient list that could have come out a chemistry textbook, have crossed a threshold where the word food no longer applies.

If they aren't foods, what are they? They're drugs without benefits. They have no nutritional value, but still affect blood chemistry. They're impostors disguised in the costumes of food. In the eyes of cellular intelligence, a potato chip is the equivalent of plastic. And because such impostors are not food, the cell's resulting confusion would be similar to that of Greek children taking an exam in Spanish. Test failures would be due to design error, not to the children.

To switch metaphors, the cells respond to processed food as they would to hostile forces. Chemicals and processed foods are, in your body's opinion, the enemy. After identifying them as invaders, the cells mobilize defenses to neutralize them. And this work is done through scavengers called free radicals. The host is quite the fundamentalist in this regard, sending the free radicals to attack anything it doesn't recognize as friendly forces. Flush with its aggressive powers, the army can begin attacking its own countrymen. And when this occurs, a form of degeneration at the cellular level has begun.

The standard American diet, sometimes called SAD, is full of factory-machined foods. Much of the contents of the plastic, tin, and cardboard containers in the average supermarket should be tossed into the dumpster. If you care for your friends, don't give them cookies during the holidays. Why give them an unhealthy gift? And if you receive well-intentioned holiday sweets, you're better off throwing them into the garbage after your friends have gone home with your warm thanks and your basket of fruit. I thought of this one day as I carried leftover Halloween candy to a home across the street with six kids—I realized I needed to redefine neighborhood friendliness.

The more we tamper with the natural architecture of a food, the less likely our cells will recognize it. In contrast, a big salad of leafy greens, yellow peppers, cherry tomatoes, purple olives, bright white onions, and red sockeye salmon is an understandable language for communicating with the mettle of the universe sleeping in our cells. Whole foods are living forces, not substances, that link the acumen of the natural world with the power nascent in the human cell.

Mystics might have said that when we eat a salad, the world is nurturing itself at one particular spot. In this transpersonal view, eating, or any action for that matter, is never just an individual, isolated event. It's simply the whole, the Whole, showing up in particular shapes and colors at one physical location. While a salad may be a collection of antioxidants in gainful service of our physiological needs, it's also the poetry of the world resonating with the rhythm of life bringing itself alive. Like a good rhyme scheme, it creates cadence in the body. It links the body to the ethos of nature, preparing us in a fitting prelude for the integration of our souls into nature's wisdom. To eat healthily is to be resonant with the splendor and the authority of nature's sagacity, just as sails in concert with the wind help a yacht glide across the sea.

The chasm between knowing and doing

For many people, the real health challenge is doing what they already know to be healthy. Most, especially those who would read this kind of book, already know the basics of good nutrition. During my lectures, I've never seen anyone look startled to hear that vegetables and fruit are healthy for you. While the U.S. could use a massive policy initiative to educate the public about nutrition, the roadblock for many people is not knowing, but doing. We already know that cakes, pies, sodas, fries, donuts, and candies are not health foods and that ketchup is not a vegetable. But it's hard to buck old habits that have us pinned to the floor like a hapless wrestler. Many mature, sensible, educated adults find themselves feeble under the spell cast by desserts, sugar, alcohol, sodas, and diet sodas. While a trickle of these substances won't hurt, a steady stream will.

Many of us will often need months, or years, of effort to reshape the landscape of our diets. For some, the switch can be easy. But for many others, reducing or eliminating ice cream, cake, and cookies can be as excruciating as kicking an addiction in rehab. For those drinking five or six diet sodas daily, which is not uncommon, change comes hard. I was surprised when I first encountered the Herculean grip that diet sodas can have on people. Fruit and vegetables often feel like penalties or the brainchild of a masochist for those accustomed to burgers, pizzas, and the fast food menu. For all those trying to eat better, note that when Jack LaLanne said, "If man made it, don't eat it," he wasn't suggesting that cookies and cakes were permissible if baked by Mom.

Escaping from the grip of an indulgent culture and breaking the shackles of entrenched habit is one of American society's great health challenges. And an opportunity. When we think of the healthcare crisis, we usually think of economic, political, and policy matters. They're all parts of the dilemma, and we certainly need efforts devoted to solving them. But one huge, unrecognized challenge for the American public is to leap across the chasm between knowing and doing.

Change slowly

Improving nutrition habits can present unique challenges for each person, but a few hints may be helpful here. While a few people can switch to a healthy diet overnight through a mere act of will, rapid changes more often follow the diagnosis of a life-threatening illness. Even then, some people will find it hard to change. Often, change must come gradually. Our taste buds are demanding, impetuous, and forever discontent, set in their ways like an old grandpa. A good dosage of time may be necessary to redirect their drift. At first, a little discipline might be needed to resist the hypnotic music emanating from the ice cream in the freezer and the brownies in the pantry. The taste buds may be reluctant or obstinate when first switching to a diet with more whole foods. But eventually, the body's natural inclination to be healthy will kick in, and eating whole foods will become habitual. Eating healthy need not be a white-knuckle effort forever, as taste buds can eventually come to find processed foods, or at least the queasy consequences of eating them, unpleasant.

If the thought of eating better sets off a barroom brawl in your mind, you might start by setting a goal that's so small and simple that you'll be sure to succeed. For example, rather than starting off with the goal of eating a salad every day, you might try for just one more salad during the week. By first keeping your standards at ground level, but with a bona fide commitment to your goal, success is more likely. The sense of accomplishment gives you a spark with its small but encouraging glimmer of success. In this case, the emotional boost of small triumphs is more important than the size of the task. This works with exercise as well, as I've seen many patients turn timid beginnings into a robust exercise program. Sometimes a commitment to exercise for just ten minutes in a week is enough to get them going on a more substantial regimen. So it's the glint and glow of small successes that motivate us, not the size of the goal. For those who are wholly inert, just getting started is of key importance.

It also helps to remember that your diet doesn't need to be perfect. It's close to impossible any way, and goals too lofty can be a prelude to failure and discouragement. Since the human body can forgive like a saint, it can handle a few chemicals or insulin spikes here and there, even the occasional deep-fried Twinkie. Most people my age spent their early school years eating lunches of white-bread baloney sandwiches, dyed sugar drinks, sodas, potato chips, and candy, and during the summers, we ate popsicles that turned our eager tongues green, orange, or purple with chemical food dyes. But we managed, as the body can rebound from such insults. However, to be clear, the average American diet is now toxic.

What I'm addressing is the other end of the spectrum: the frustrations that always come on the heels of an all-or-nothing approach to eating healthy. When people stumble just once after starting on a healthier path, they'll often toss out the whole effort and engorge themselves on sweet fatty rewards. But when our nutritional regimen allows for the occasional indulgence, we can persist far more easily. Some people are caught in a compulsive obsession about health foods. Eating in fear and compulsion is itself unhealthy.

For most of my patients, I discourage the notion of a perfect diet. Instead, I usually suggest that, at the minimum, they set their standards at eating healthily enough to see signs of progress. A health regimen should be at least rigorous enough to tip us forward, to show some signs of progress in weight, vitality, and overall wellbeing, however minor. While an ultrapure diet is ideal, especially for those with serious illnesses, it often means too much pressure, time, or work for most of us. If, instead, you're eating about 80 to 90 percent healthy, that may be enough to tip you forward.

Some patients have said that once I suggested they not eat the perfect diet, they lost weight for the first time in their lives. Until then, deviating from their diet would lead first to discouragement and then to abandonment of their goals. An intentionally imperfect nutrition plan could, for example, schedule an occasional small portion of a rich dessert to reduce the pressure. For most people, the difference between one piece of cake a week and none is negligible; but cake or dessert every night is a 700 percent increase and another matter entirely. The relaxed, natural drift of eating healthily can take time to cultivate, and once in place, it can be effortless. In fact, the foods that used to tempt you might one day look appalling. As a recovered sugarholic, I'll attest to that. And it helps to remember that the full chorus of nature's power is behind you on this.

The essence of nourishment

Whole foods do more than issue smart instructions to our bodies. They help restore our relationship to the natural order of the world. They make us intimate with the fecundity of soil and water, with the muscle of forest and mountain. We've seen in previous chapters how a broader definition of health includes our relationship to the world and to others, as well as respect for the customs of the universe. Similarly, the ingestion of whole foods helps us become better citizens of the world as anima mundi. By fulfilling our civic duties at the cellular level, we do so, by extension, at cosmic levels.

We can think of eating whole foods as an act of reverence, a bow to the wisdom that created miracles like corn and peas, an activity that helps us live in the depths of our awareness instead of on the surface tensions of a culture that puts panache before substance.

Good nourishment helps us move with the rhymes and rhythms of the earth's intelligence, whether we see that as improved neurochemical function or as an act of artistry. The mind, just like the body, depends on the vital effusions of the earth—the body is never only physical until it's dead. Eating whole foods, then, is a way of honoring both the provenance and the future of our spiritual selves.

Water

Water plays a crucial role in the sinuous aliveness of the earth. The rains, rivers, and oceans within the human body are, as the Native Americans said, the lifeblood of the planet. Without it, there is no field or forest, bird or wolf. Just as the body's blood transports information and supplies, water is part of the communication system both in the human body and on the planet. Water is the juice of life itself, the matrix of organic origins, revered in ancient cultures as a gift from the heavens. But unfortunately, our frantic, bloated schedules can numb us to the subtle signals from the body asking for hydration.

Research on how much water we need has been mixed. Some recent studies have suggested that we don't need the proverbial eight glasses a day. But some researchers insist that drinking plenty of pure, fresh water is necessary. Despite these mixed messages, or perhaps because of them, it's helpful to learn for ourselves what our bodies need, to listen closely to the whispers of thirst. Since each body is different, the need for water will vary. In Chinese medicine, we can get clues to a body's need for water, as well as its overall condition, from a diagnosis of the tongue. The tongue is a trove of information on the internal condition of the body, and it can be bluish, purplish, reddish, pink, or pale. Each color points to different sets of physiological imbalances, a subject too complex to summarize here. In this scheme, for example, a dry, reddish tongue is an indication of too much "fire" and heat, and therefore, in part, not enough water.

A good experiment would be to drink six to eight glasses of water, or even more, every day for two or three weeks and watch for any subtle changes. You can repeat the experiment several times to better understand its effects.

Nutrition and prevention

Nourishing ourselves well is crucial for preventing, or at least delaying, the breakdown of the body. An ancient Chinese text, *The Yellow Emperor's Classic of Internal Medicine*, states that treating a disease after it has struck is like digging a well after getting thirsty. Eating whole foods and exercising well to prevent illness is smart beyond measure—they are elongated levers of health. They help us avoid medications, surgeries, and hospitalizations that can cost hundreds of thousands of dollars. They help us be productive and meaningfully engaged in our work. They can prevent the descent into hell that disease can bring to our lives, and decrease the chances of our families and friends enduring the ordeal of seeing us sick and then becoming exhausted from taking care of us.

The physical and emotional stresses of caring for an ailing spouse or parent can be a health risk for the caregiver. In my practice, I've often seen how the patient becomes symptomatic not during the caretaking, but a few months after it's over. The shingles, the back pain, the shoulder pain, the heart problems—the caregiver didn't have time for these while nursing the sick spouse for a year. A bigger job demanded her attention. Only after it's all over is there enough time and space to let the body reset its communication systems to signal distress. Preventing all this is a bargain in every way imaginable.

The basic requisites for health are similar, if not identical, no matter what the disease. Whether it's for the prevention of fatigue, anxiety, depression, heart disease, diabetes, cancer, Alzheimer's, bowel problems, PMS, and so on, exercise and good nourishment help.

When well nourished, your body is like a garden overflowing with spring flowers. Or for those with a more mechanical bent, an exotic sports car with premium fuel. If everyone were nourished well enough, the number of preventable chronic diseases would plummet. And since the cost of treating chronic diseases forms the bulk of our national healthcare bill, this is no small matter. Although a well-nourished and exercised body is not all that's needed, since illness often comes from a combination of influences, it's a substantial contribution to anyone's quality of life.

Exercise and motion

In the way we've looked at nutrition as nourishment, we can also think of the essence of exercise as motion. Since I have never met a person who didn't already know that exercise is good for you, I will focus on its essence.

Virtually every patient will admit, with a slight tenor of guilt, to needing more exercise. As with eating whole foods, the core issue for most people is not the need for more information, but just doing it, just getting the fingers to lace up those running shoes. Few of us need to be told that exercise will help us feel healthier and more alive, and we already know that the first and most important exercise is leaping across the chasm of inertia. What more do we need to know about exercise that will get us out of the lounger? The thought of exercise can leave us reluctant or petulant—sentiments made clear by Robert Hutchins, who wrote, "Whenever I feel like exercise, I lie down until the feeling passes."

Motion

With regard to exercise, we can redefine it as the motion of life itself. First, let's look at motion in its broadest sense. For the body, we can think of motion as a measure of aliveness. The more you can move about, the more fit you are. The body's ability to stretch, run, and bend is a sign of life.

Next, we have motion within the body, and that includes the lungs breathing, the heart beating, the blood circulating.

Further yet, motion occurs at the cellular level as the transport of nutrients from the bloodstream into the cells, the packaging of nutrients into energy bonds, the elimination of waste through the cell walls, and the docking of good-mood neurochemicals like serotonin, endorphin, and dopamine at their receptors in the brain like yachts docking at the marina. All of it is motion.

Conversely, the end of motion is the end of life. When movement stops—in the eyes, the breath, the swishing of blood through the arteries, the electrical pulsing in the brain—then we're no longer alive. So the capacity to move is a characteristic of the living.

Beyond physical movement, we have its psychological and spiritual analogues. To move about on the playing fields of creativity and innovation, to have a thought enter and exit the mind, to expand the boundaries of consciousness itself: all this is motion as an expression of what the ancients called the life force.

As we redefine physical exercise in its essence, we can see it as a way to align ourselves with a core imperative of being alive. To exercise is to go in its abstracted sense, an idea resonant with the search for essence through abstractionism in the arts. We saw this with painters like Rothko, Pollock, Kandinsky, and de Kooning, who, with their contemporaries, worked to grasp the essence behind the visible world. Initially, they'd all learned to paint the realistic form and color of a human face, but then they became curious about how to paint the spirits behind the face.

In a similar sense, to *go* is to voyage through our lives: to breathe, laugh, earn, learn, and to pursue a fulfilling, meaningful life. All that's familiar to us about exercise—its great benefits for the heart, brain, immune system, lungs, circulation, blood sugar control, and so on—is only part of the picture. Playing tennis and riding a bike are not just "physical" activities. They're mind-body activities. Once again, we're redefining what we normally consider to be purely physical as something equally psychological, existential, and spiritual.

It's catalytic

Referring again to methods that substitute, control, or catalyze, exercise is catalytic. It doesn't just polish or tweak the body. It transforms it in the same alchemical way a child struggling with second grade math can grow into a professor, statesman, or billionaire. Exercise has that capacity to transform us at the cellular level as well as in the shape of our bodies. It's not just a state change, like turning a light switch on and off, or changing a feeling from bad to good. Instead, it turns the lead of fatigue into the gold of vitality, meek potential into roaring actualization, a seed into bright red roses. While medieval physical alchemy led only to dead ends, a true alchemy is found in the transformative potential of mind and body.

An analogy for the catabolic and anabolic effects of exercise is given by Chris Crowley and Henry Lodge, M.D., in their book, *Younger Next Year*. First, exercise destroys muscle cells with inflammation by producing a substance called cytokine-6. This is similar to the way a contractor must first rip up your kitchen before he begins remodeling. Before he installs the new cabinets and counters, he first destroys and dismantles. Next, the cytokine-6 automatically brings about the production of cytokine-10, a substance that repairs and remodels the cells. The result is a new, attractive kitchen, or in the body, a new set of muscles and more. When you see a muscle start to bulge after a few months of weight training, it's not the old muscle getting bigger. It's fresh new muscle tissue that hadn't existed before. Exercise can literally remodel the body.

One notable benefit of exercise is that it can increase the number of mitochondria in each cell. Mitochondria perform the job of bundling nutrients into clusters of potential energy known as adenosine triphosphate, or ATP. These clusters burn like gasoline in a car engine to propel the body. When we exercise and get in shape, we create more mitochondria. And the more we have, the more energy we have for deepening our relationships, for earning an income, for walking our spiritual path—and for lacing up those running shoes.

The cycle of destruction and creation here is a parallel to what I wrote in the chapter on health as transformation, where we saw the storms and cyclones of our lives as catalysts for growth. We saw that the ogres plaguing the hero's journey are necessary for our development. Similarly, remodeling both body and mind starts with creative destruction. The stress of movement—whether in running, swimming, dancing, or weight training—renovates the cellular landscape in our limbs and in our brains.

Designed to move

Just as the human body is designed to flourish with the ingestion of natural foods, it is also designed to do so through motion. During the millions of years it took for the human body to become what it is today, it was almost always on the move. To find food and shelter, we spent about four hours a day climbing, running, digging, or hunting. On the yardstick of human evolution, the amount of time we've had a sedentary lifestyle takes up about 4/1000 of an inch, a measure so small it can't be seen by the naked eye.

This historical backdrop supports the more recent and abundant research pointing to a sedentary life as a contributor to obesity and illness. Since we're designed to move, a life of idleness doesn't belong in evolution's rulebook. By exercising, we respect the legacy of motion going back millions of years. We must move. It's both our birthright and imperative.

Exercise is essential for our children as well, and lucky for them, and not so lucky for the tired mother, they can't stop moving. But all that motion helps produce new brain cells: when a toddler is jumping and dancing, she's growing new neurons and a bigger, better brain. Exercise promotes both neurogenesis, the production of new brain cells, and neuroplasticity, the rewiring of the brain to do new jobs.

For adults and children both, prolonged exercise in the form of, say, thirty minutes at 80–90 percent of maximum heart rate five times a week can stimulate the production of BDNF (brain derived neurotrophic factor) in the brain. BDNF is a building block for new brain cells. And the more we have, the faster and smarter our brains. One example of exercise's potential effects can be found in the success of a school district in Illinois.

In lieu of the usual sports-oriented physical education programs, Naperville District 203 created a program emphasizing fitness. Students exercised daily before the start of classes, aiming for heart rates of 80–90 percent of maximum while using a heart-rate monitor. As a result, and with no curriculum changes, academic scores improved dramatically. During one year, the scores on standardized tests placed their eighth-graders first in the world in science and sixth in math, whereas American students as a whole ranked eighteenth and nineteenth, respectively. Research by the California Department of Education has found that on academic tests, students who are physically fit consistently and significantly outperform those who are not.

Moving your body in novel ways and increasing your heart rate, whether through gymnastics, dance, basketball, or yoga, rewires the brain. The brain can be rewired to learn even those skills you thought were beyond reach. When a violin player practices for years, the part of the brain governing the left hand grows much bigger. And although in our later years the potential for growing new brain cells is reduced, it doesn't vanish entirely. We can still rewire the old brain to learn new tricks as it gets older. The essence of motion, then, is not just mindless physical activity, but a creative force that awakens possibilities.

One middle-aged patient of mine had minor, recurring problems, including sinusitis, for which she'd come to see me every few months. Though her diet was good, and though she was healthy overall and fairly fit, she didn't like to exercise. Then suddenly, she decided to start training for marathons. Before long, she was running up to forty miles a week and completing one or two marathons a year. It greatly improved her strength and resilience.

In her mid-fifties, Paula came occasionally for the support of her overall wellness. One day, after I'd been treating her at regular but infrequent intervals for several years, she started taking lessons in ballroom dancing. Instantly, she was enthralled with the romantic moods and beauty of dancing. And soon, her entire life changed as it began to revolve around her new pursuit. Within a few months, her outlook on her life and the condition of her body improved markedly. A lingering mistrust of men dissolved after many safe and enchanting times in their arms; she was happier and more energetic. And with a spiritual exuberance and freedom of motion she'd never known before, she lost weight, felt effervescent, and found her self-esteem strengthened.

New standards

So how much should you exercise? Here's one possible standard: more than you think is reasonable.

In 1973, my friends and I got directions from a camper to an obscure but magnificent spot in Colorado's Dinosaur National Monument. After describing a few turns, he told us we'd get on a steep, rocky road. And then when we felt horribly lost, we'd be right on track. As we drove into the desolate landscape and along the poorly marked road, we felt completely disoriented at times. Then we remembered his words, and continued, reassured. It was precisely the guideline we used to find our way across the wilderness neverland to the towering cliff standing watch over the green river. Similarly, by today's standards, the right amount of exercise may seem wrong, or oddly excessive. An exercise regimen appropriate today is one that a few decades ago might have had our neighbors calling us health nuts. The well-respected Institute of Medicine recommends one hour a day of moderate exercise like walking, or a half-hour a day of vigorous exercise like running. With mountains of research on the impact of motion on health, the bar has been raised.

Keeping the body well nourished with whole foods and keeping it in motion are essential if body and mind are to thrive. Motion and nourishment help us resist all manner of disease and symptoms: inflammation, obesity, cancer, Alzheimer's, heart disease, depression, anxiety, insomnia, diabetes, immune system disorders, and virtually any illness. Motion and nourishment are highly placed archangels of health.

Many studies have suggested that exercise increases longevity by at least several years. But beyond any quantitative benefits, it also changes the flavor of life. To this point, many elderly patients tell me they're not afraid of death. Instead, they're afraid of being helpless and in pain as their bodies slide toward death. They'll take short and happy over prolonged and wretched.

One patient of mine, who started treatments with me when he was eighty years old, came for a treatment every week of every year, except for occasional snow days or vacations, for fourteen straight years. The typical schedule for a patient in my practice is about once a week for six to eight weeks, after which we taper off at a rate depending on their progress. After the initial series, many people like to come every four to eight weeks for health enhancement. But this gentleman was resolved to come far more often. I was occasionally stressed by the routine of treating him week after week, year after year, when it wasn't needed. To be honest, it became boring for me. But I didn't have the heart to deny him his wishes. To my insistence that he didn't need to come so often, he insisted harder that he did. The reason? When it was his time to die, he wanted to go quickly and painlessly in his sleep. Over the years, he must have told me at least thirty times in his hoary voice, "When I die, Doc, I just want to go quick." By being in the best shape possible with weekly acupuncture, he hoped to increase the chances of dying without fanfare. Above all, he didn't want to vegetate, to burden his family, to be salivating in a wheelchair. One cold winter night, when he was ninety-four, he died instantly in his sleep as he had wished.

A well-conditioned body can help with a vibrant life now, and reduce suffering later toward the end of our lives. Remembering Helen Klein, Jack LaLanne, and spritely centenarians might help us recalibrate our notions of what we consider age-appropriate exercise.

The pursuit of health as a moral act

We have a steady stream of research splashed on the front pages of all our media touting the health benefits of good nutrition and abundant exercise. We know now that a good exercise regimen and whole foods help you live longer, feel happier, be smarter, be more energetic, and be less likely to get sick. But here's another reason to take good care of your body, one that seems to take many people off guard: people love you.

A "you" is made meaningful in context. And that context includes a social web of friends, family, and community, an idea expressed in the African concept of ubuntu made popular by Nelson Mandela and Archbishop Desmond Tutu. What usually doesn't occur to us is that when we're sick, this social network as a whole is made symptomatic. Because your spouse, partner, parents, children, and friends love you, your illness affects them deeply. They can become exhausted from taking care of you and taking up the slack at home, beleaguered enough to be at greater risk of becoming sick themselves.

The notion of rugged individualism is by now a cliché of the American pioneering spirit. It certainly has been a driving force in the extraordinary growth the country has seen since 1776. But the merits of individualism can obscure holism, our relatedness to loved ones and community, ubuntu, our being one flower in a garden of relationships. Existentially, we can't not be related. As we then look at our health in all the contexts of our lives, it clearly affects the lives of others. If we're sick and can't get to work, colleagues may need to assume some of our work. If we stay home, somebody must spend time taking care of us, sometimes until depleted.

If you're starting to feel guilty here, note that feeling guilt or shame is both optional and unproductive. A better response would be one consistent with the point being made here: taking excellent care of our bodies can be the expression of a compassionate responsibility toward our loved ones. It can come from the recognition that a fit, happy, and healthy you is a handsome gift to others, a non-random act of kindness. You'll be better able to nurture family and friends in all ways. As we saw earlier, George Leonard and Michael Murphy asserted that the pursuit of health, when we can see ourselves as part of the Whole, is a moral act.

Our fondness for individualism, flavored by a culture of indulgence, can lead to the axiom that the freedom to indulge is an inalienable right. In the framework of our Constitution, that's true. But the right to indulge is based on the understandable but slightly askew notion that pleasure equals happiness. It almost feels like a hard-earned, God-given, well-deserved, Constitutional right to drink all I want, eat all the dessert I want, and do as little exercise as I please.

An entirely different view is that our health is a deposit into the accounts of our loved ones, and our illness a withdrawal. As long as we're healthy, we're capable of supporting and loving those around us. We're able-bodied enough to contribute our talents to them and to the world. But when we're sick, our loved ones are weighted with worry and the world is deprived of our gifts. It isn't egotism to know that people love you and that your illness can unsettle their souls. On the contrary, denial of this can be a form of reverse egotism.

Year after year, I've listened to people trampled by the news that a family member has been diagnosed with a serious illness. Often, the news hits the loved ones harder than it does the patient. The patient is resolved at the prospect of impending death, while the spouse is berserk with grief and anxiety. One act of kindness toward your loved ones would be to sculpt a healthy body, even while struggling with the anesthesia induced by a culture of indulgence. When you become fit and healthy, you're taking out spiritual insurance and increasing the chances that the generosity of your soul will be more durable and available longer to those who need it most.

Hear the breathing

As we've said, whole foods are the flesh of the earth. They help reconnect us to our true nature, allowing us access to the powers in wind, fire, earth, wood, and water. They are literally a bite taken out of the physical universe that we ingest, digest, and then convert, ultimately, into the human drama. When we eat, we ingest not just food, but its quintessence and mystery as well. Real food, whole food, is a miracle drug that can nurture, support, and heal every system in the body.

Exercise also is a miracle drug. It makes all systems healthier. Good food and exercise, matched to the condition and needs of each person, can amplify the effects of the services you receive from health professionals, and in some cases, can reverse problems beyond the grasp of professional interventions.

When we eat healthily, we nourish the endless pregnancy in our minds, bodies, and souls. We extract the potential for vitality, which, for working purposes, is best considered infinite.

Underneath the greens, reds, and yellows of food, and the sweat of a workout, we'll find a hymn of possibility, a canto of wisdom. We can look at nourishment and motion through the usual lens of metabolic dynamics. But for a less mechanistic view, we can also consider them poetry, as in the Japanese Shinto tradition that pays homage to the spirits known as kami that lie breathing in the wood and water, earth and stone, rice and onion. Kami are no less invisible to the naked eye than molecules. This is resonant with the Native American view expressed by Zitkala Sa when she said the Great Spirit speaks through the rippling of the waters and the sweet breathing of flowers. The rippling and breathing are not sound and scent, but incantations. This is similar, if not identical, to one of Plato's lasting contributions to philosophy in which he saw that these spirits, which he called forms or ideals, are shapes of truth hiding behind the physical appearance of the world. What our eyes can see is just the costume of those truths. When eating whole foods, we can remember the kami.

The challenge in softening the analytical, mechanistic view of the world and of the human body is to look past the surface glare into the hidden underbelly of things. If we stood on a Colorado lakeshore looking at the blue waters, we could see H_2O, the color blue—or a reflection of mystery. If we gaze with a clear, silent mind, with a bit of luck, the doors of perception may open wide to show us the heavens invisible to everyday eyes. While the muffled presence of this mystery and its magnificence is easier to detect in the forest and ocean, it's also there in equal measure in the steel and concrete canyons of cities, which are no less a part of the Whole than the most pristine flower in the wilderness. In the end, we can understand eating and exercising as spiritual acts.

While knowing about the benefits of nutrition and exercise can help motivate us, we can also find inspiration by remembering the bigger picture: healthy eating and exercise help restore the ethos of nature's wisdom to our lives. They grant us the suppleness of water, the passion of fire, the might of trees, the fecundity of earth, and the speed of the wind. They help us take one small step forward in dispelling our illusions of separateness by keeping the mind one bit clearer and the heart one bit softer. To echo the phrasing of the mystics, the whole universe presents itself to us in that one deep breath, that one bite of avocado, that one sip of cool water.

The act of eating, in this view, is how the universe keeps itself alive through us, propagating its wisdom. At the very least, it's the evolutionary drive of the biological self that seeks to keep life going. The very essence of evolution, the intelligence guiding the transformation of the human experience, takes place right there at the taste bud when we eat, at those few square centimeters where the bean and broccoli touch the tongue. The enormity of the whole can show up as a hologram in the most microcosmic of places.

Eating whole foods and exercising are foundations for our psychological and spiritual growth. If those foundations are shaky, so goes the work of becoming fully ourselves. If they're strong, we flourish and help the world, if only one other human being at a time. We are healthier when we hear the sweet breathing of flowers.

Chapter Eight

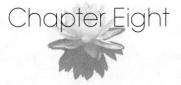

The Whole

Holistic medicine is an approach that treats the whole person. While that may seem like a vague idea, it's vital for understanding the essence of health and healing. Treating the whole person is a notion still scarce in clinical medicine, but it's of great consequence, representing a marked difference between the integrative and conventional approaches to healing. In recent years, the word terrain has sometimes been used to describe what we call the whole in integrative medicine, and while it's not as accurate, it's more tangible. I will use both interchangeably.

Much of what I've already written points to the value of seeing the whole picture. The broken window story shows how we must include the big picture if we are to understand why the glass keeps breaking. That's a whole. With that in mind, we can see that the path to either health or illness is not a single line like a hiking trail to the summit. Instead, it's more a mixture like soup or a blended fruit drink.

One central part of the idea of the whole is that everything is connected to everything. Unfortunately, that can lead to mind-numbing vastness and ambiguity. It's admittedly a nebulous idea. But the solution to the ambiguity is to pinpoint those relevant connections that give us leverage for change. In the broken window story, for example, we can focus on the way the parents' psychological and physical health affects the son's behavior. But we don't need to focus on the grandparents, as their influence on present conditions is too remote. Knowing what to include as relevant is an art.

As we consider what it means to speak of a whole, we can look at it from the broadest possible philosophical view. In that case, it becomes appropriate to capitalize it and name it the Whole, capital W, which includes everything imaginable.

To start looking at this essential relatedness, I'll recount a brief conversation I had with physicist Dr. Hans Peter Duerr, a former colleague of one of the most influential physicists in history, Nobel Prize winner Werner Heisenberg.

> The universe is not a world of separate things and events, of external spectators and an impersonal spectacle. It is an integral whole.
>
> – Ervin Laszlo

Dr. Duerr was in Baltimore at a Johns Hopkins conference on bridging the gaps between conventional and holistic views of medicine. After he finished his lecture on how quantum physics helps us see the world differently, I walked up to him to ask a question. He looked the part of genius scientist with thick glasses, wild hair, worn blazer, and flashing eyes. I said, "I can hardly believe my ears, so I wanted to make sure I heard you correctly. Are you really saying that in quantum physics, the fundamental building block of the universe is no longer the subatomic particle, but relationship itself?" With eyes flashing even brighter and an excited grin, he answered with a resounding "Yes." If Martin Buber had been there, he might have smiled at how this resonated with his own words, "In the beginning was the relation."

Along similar lines, the Oxford physicist Vtlatko Vedral argues that the smallest parts of physical reality are not subatomic particles, or waves, or vibrating "strings" of energy.

He says the smallest units in the universe are information, parallel to the idea in nutrigenomics that food is information. So, scientifically speaking, our bodies aren't made of matter. Instead, they're made of, well, clouds—though even that is still too mechanistic a metaphor given the subtleties in quantum physics.

Some sort of metaphor seems appropriate when the literal scientific truth is that our bodies are made of information and relationship. If it's confusing, it's not a deficit on your part. We're still drawn to thinking that apples are made of atomic bits though the idea that has been outdated in physics for nearly a century. The idea that matter is made of information doesn't negate the old atomistic view of things. It just goes a step further.

In today's world, then, *relationship* and *information* have replaced atoms as constituents of matter. Apples, trucks, and elephants are made of Relationship, not atoms. While this might sound like lunacy, this is straight from the penthouses of quantum physics.

Transferring this idea to the realm of human experience helps us see the body anew, to see that it's more like water than earth, more like air than stone. Being able to grasp that idea, if only in good faith, helps us understand those healing methods that see the human body as energy with a shape.

> The most fundamental phenomenon in the universe is relationship.
>
> –Jonas Salk

Acupuncture, homeopathy, Healing Touch, qi gong, Reiki, and other energy manipulation techniques can induce changes that would be baffling to those who see the human body as a collection of biological bits. Most of these techniques work on the premise that the human body is a form of energy, which is a little like saying it's made of electricity. But this doesn't negate the biological view of the body or its astonishing discoveries. Bioenergy happens to be one of the body's unseen dimensions, while biological form is visible. And while quantum physics doesn't explain why these holistic therapies work, its bizarre and outlandish discoveries help the mind stay receptive to the worlds beyond the orbit of mechanistic science.

My intention is not to present an airtight case about wholeness, but to have the idea become a practical force for change in your life. Both instinct and culture have taught us to focus on the symptom, the part, the squeaky wheel. But thinking of the Whole in addition to the part can improve your chances of becoming or staying healthy.

An idea not so strange

We're already acquainted with the saying that the whole is greater than the sum of its parts. But that doesn't define a whole, or the Whole. The idea is vague enough that we risk getting lost in ambiguities. Fortunately, the idea of a whole is not at all foreign to our everyday thinking.

The words *society* and *forest*, for example, refer to wholes. We see cars and stores, people and houses, but there is no separate and discrete thing called society. We can't touch a society. Similarly, we can touch a pine or a birch, but we can never touch a thing called forest. Nor can we put a finger on intelligence, as no part of the brain contains any physical substance called intelligence.

The brain is not intelligence but a chunk of gray fatty matter. We won't find intelligence anywhere in the neurons, the basic units of the brain, or the synapses between them. Nor does a gene for intelligence exist. Neurons send signals to each other so we can think and feel, but that's not intelligence either. So the twist is that no intelligence exists in the human brain (insert favorite joke here) because the word refers to only an observer's opinion about a person's abilities.

Proof of intelligence comes in the form of an A on a test, an award, a Nobel Prize, or other measures, but these are social yardsticks, assessments in the mind of an observer. They're smoking-gun evidence. If a person is accurate, insightful, and capable, then we say she has intelligence. But it's not a thing we find in the brain.

Then there's love, which also doesn't exist according to scientific measures. We can't point to a single, measurable thing and say this is *love*. People lust for it, kill for it, and die for it, but we can't see it on a microscope slide. Love, the core of human existence, the energy that makes the world go round, is indefinable and immeasurable. We have no double-blind randomized controlled clinical trials to prove it exists.

All this may help explain why we must talk about a Whole in medicine. This opaque notion, like love and intelligence or forest and society, is ambiguous and mysterious but of great consequence.

As patients receive treatments such as acupuncture, massage, homeopathy, or naturopathy, they often feel better overall—a pervasive feeling that's different from the sensations of a particular symptom. Most people will say it's hard to describe, but in some indefinable way they feel better in total. It's hard to describe precisely because the feeling is so broad and non-specific. Given the ambiguities, it's understandable that people struggle to find the words for it.

In contrast, a high blood pressure reading or a low potassium level is objective, specific, and measurable. But overall wellbeing is subjective, nonspecific, and therefore immeasurable. The four objective vital signs in medicine are the pulse rate, blood pressure, the rate of breathing, and body temperature. Some hospitals include pain as the fifth. But a patient's overall subjective sense of wellbeing should be the sixth because it's an important reflection of health. While it's not foolproof, it's often a good measure of our internal condition.

So how do we better understand what this means in health and healing? I'll explain further with stories of my patients, starting with Caroline.

I ache all over. And I feel wonderful.

If a voice could smile, Caroline's did. She was retired, dividing her time between working for a flower shop and babysitting her grandchildren. She came to me hoping that acupuncture would help with arthritic pains in her joints. Though her medications were helping, she was still in pain.

After a few weeks of acupuncture, she was responding better than I'd expected. During each weekly visit, she said her pains were improving slightly. Progress was slow, but at least the trend was positive. Then one day, Caroline came in for her fifth session and said that because she'd been feeling better, she decided on her own to stop taking all her arthritis medications. Medical decisions like this should have been made with her doctor, so I was surprised. When I asked how she felt, she answered with a comment I've never forgotten—it encapsulates the difference between the whole and the part. With her usual big grin, she said, "I ache all over. And I feel wonderful."

During the following months, Caroline continued to improve. While she never became completely free of pain, she felt markedly better and no longer needed arthritis medications. But most importantly, she felt well overall. She felt the pep, the verve, the goodness of being alive.

Carl was a retired, seventy-three-year-old businessman who came to me with severe pain in his ankles and shoulders. His doctors had also diagnosed a pain in his left foot as shingles, a painful inflammation triggered by the chicken pox virus. Many patients have said it's the worst pain they've ever experienced. For his other pains, Carl had gotten three steroid injections, disc surgery, a nerve block, and medications. For the shingles, he'd gotten medications as well. But the pains persisted.

After two acupuncture treatments, the pain in his shoulder was gone. After four treatments, so went the pain in his ankles. But the shingles in his foot hadn't budged. In the meantime, Carl was pleased with his progress and was becoming more animated, more vibrant overall. While the disappearance of some of his pain was welcome news, those were *particulars*. I was also watching for improvements in the terrain, his overall health, the *whole*. This was essential for the long-term and for the big picture because he had diabetes and high blood pressure. If he was getting healthier overall, that might help his other illnesses and steer his entire life in a better direction.

One day, he came in for his appointment and told me he was getting stronger. While on the golf course the day before, he was able to open bottles of drinking water, something he'd been unable to do before. Even better, his golf swing had gotten stronger. While improving at golf and opening water bottles might not sound like significant clinical markers, they were representations of important changes in the whole. They were pointing to broader physiological changes. Carl's terrain was improving. You could see it in his livelier eyes, hear it in his stronger voice, and notice it in his body's new vigor. These are important clinical considerations, as the absence of pain is insufficient for real vitality and integration. For many patients, that overall sense of vitality must come first before particular symptoms improve.

At that point, I trusted that Carl was healing at the roots. He wasn't healing completely, but the changes were coming from the bottom up. Nothing was being numbed or blunted or suppressed by acupuncture. Carl also worked to decrease his intake of cookies, ice cream, starchy carbs, and processed foods. With my encouragement, he started to restore his long lost friendship with vegetables.

It's rare for a technique in integrative medicine to silence the signals, to turn off the smoke alarm. Instead, when it works by strengthening the whole, the very pedigree of the symptom is being erased. A symptom treated by a catalytic method improves because it's healing from the inside out, from the roots on up. The change comes from catalyzing, not substituting. The symptom is not blanketed and then hidden in the cellar. An overall boost in a person's quality of life, how he feels in himself in total, is a good measure of authentic healing coming from the core.

Carl's case of shingles, as of this writing, continues to bother him, but with a notable difference: its impact on his life has decreased and his quality of life has improved. As we saw with Caroline, the weight of a symptom on the patient's life is an important measure of overall wellness. As in her case, Carl felt stronger and better overall, which then reduced the weight of his shingles on his mood and outlook. His angst had shrunk to mere annoyance.

Oh, by the way...

On her health questionnaire, Diane wrote that her knee pain was her main concern. An artist in her sixties, she'd had the pain since she fell off her bicycle a few months earlier. As we talked during her first few visits, I saw how she loved to talk about painting, the joy of being creative, and the meaning it brought to her life. She was so passionate about it that we spoke of little else. After her second treatment, she was pleasantly surprised to find that she was becoming a better painter. She said her paintbrush flowed more easily, ideas were coming faster, and best of all, she was creating better art.

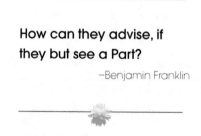

How can they advise, if they but see a Part?

—Benjamin Franklin

One day during her fourth visit, we were again talking about her art. I remember noting that neither of us had mentioned her knee pain in the last two visits. She hadn't offered any information about it, and I deliberately avoided asking her, as I wanted to see how long it would take for her to mention it again. The symptom's weight, so to speak, is often indicated by how often and how soon a patient talks about it after I walk into the room. If it stays heavy, the patient will usually mention it immediately. So I hadn't asked about her knee during the previous visit, nor had I done so in this one. Then, twenty minutes into our conversation about the thrill of art, Dianne stopped herself to say, "Oh, by the way, my knee pain is gone."

The knee pain had led her to a treatment method that helped her feel vibrant, but once she felt more creative, once her life was more colorful, the disappearance of the knee pain warranted a mere "Oh, by the way...." The pain became an afterthought, a mathematical fraction of Diane, the whole living, breathing, artful woman. What mattered most to her was the full measure of her passions. For that, a painless knee was helpful but not enough.

Here's a fourth story about the value of treating the whole.

It's time to get to work

Jason was a thirty-nine-year-old building contractor with severe, debilitating pain in his right thigh, groin, and hip resulting from a fall from a ladder. His pain had been wicked and relentless for two months. At first, he saw his primary care doctor who prescribed medications, then later an orthopedist who found no internal damage to his bones and suspected arthritis. A second orthopedist suggested a cortisone injection but Jason declined. In the meantime, Jason felt wretched, and he decided to try acupuncture. I had seen him during the previous year for other pains, but not since.

Fortunately, most of his pains were eliminated after his first acupuncture treatment, with the remainder going away after two more visits. He was, of course, thrilled that his nemesis of many months was virtually eradicated overnight. But when he expressed his satisfaction with the results, I said, "Jason, now that your pain is gone, it's time for us to get to work."

His long pause signaled that something did not compute. So I explained. Jason's terrain, his overall health, was in terrible shape. It was a wasteland.

At his age, he shouldn't have had such intense pain so long after the fall. We needed to understand the symptom's message, to drop the linear thinking that the fall off the ladder caused the pain. That would have been the equivalent of saying the baseball bat had broken the window. The whole, the big picture, included the way Jason neglected his health like the rain neglects the desert.

He was forty pounds overweight. He rarely ate vegetables or fruit, subsisting on cheese steaks, burgers, fries, and pizzas. He smoked cigarettes and drank far too much beer and soda. He smoked or ate marijuana four to five times a day, a habit he'd kept up since he was twelve—that's 49,000 times over twenty-seven years. He rarely drank water, had far too much coffee, skipped meals, ate candy bars, chips, pretzels, and cake. He never exercised. Though he would get some exercise from remodeling homes on occasion, he never got his heart rate high enough to remodel his physiology.

The twelve pulses at the wrists that acupuncturists read to assess a patient's health showed low, feeble energy. In total, his body was a toxic wasteland. It was too weak to cleanse itself—the pain's recalcitrance serving as testimony for the condition. The symptom's pedigree went back decades.

The real work

The symptom was delivering an urgent communiqué to Jason: change your life. When a person is injured, the speed of recovery will depend on his overall condition. If Jason had been fit from regular workouts and good nutrition, the injury would likely have been less severe, the recovery quicker. Now that Jason's pain was gone, we could roll up our sleeves for the real business at hand, which was to reshape the terrain. He needed a new lifestyle, an extreme physiological makeover. I suggested that biweekly acupuncture over the next six months should help—first by directly improving his physiology, and secondly by giving him a boost of energy which he could then employ for the job of carving out a whole new lifestyle, work that only he could do.

Fortunately, Jason started to take his health seriously. He cleaned up his diet, stopped smoking cigarettes, quit drinking alcohol, reduced his marijuana usage, and started taking walks. After four months and many acupuncture treatments, the big black circles under his eyes were gone and a glow had replaced the gray pallor on his face. He looked brand new. He felt more than the absence of pain, which was only occasionally aggravated by overwork. He felt good, he said. Translation: his terrain had improved.

What we want for our lives in the first place is to dance, not to trudge, and the lack of pain is only one step on the journey of a thousand smiles. If health is for something, then the absence of pain or a medical problem is itself insufficient for flourishing. There's always a next step after escaping pain or illness, and this is an essential idea in a holistic view of health. It's about more than a transition from bad to good, more than the prophylactic effects of a healthy lifestyle. It's about going from good to great.

Overall vitality is certainly not the only measure of health, nor is it foolproof. As a measure, it can be a false positive, for example, when a serious illness presents no symptom. But feeling unwell can't be a false negative. Something somewhere is amiss. It may be minor, or it may be significant like a hidden disease, but in either case, it needs your attention. As always, a medical evaluation is important for ruling out a serious condition.

Think Whole

Thinking of the Whole is an advantage in the pursuit of health because, as in Jason's case, the source of the problem is often in the Whole and not in the squeaky wheel. No single cause was behind the recalcitrance of Jason's pain. That's why integrative health practitioners focus on the entire person. This approach doesn't necessarily apply to injuries sustained in accidents or to other circumstantial conditions, but in many cases, it may be the most essential focus of treatment. On the other hand, if a patient is in otherwise excellent shape, then treating only the symptom may be reasonable.

Thinking of the whole would help Mary, who sprained her wrist falling off a chair while changing a light bulb. Appropriately, she saw her doctor who gave her medications and applied a splint. Clearly, the fall was the proximate cause. But, as Mary and I spoke at greater length, she revealed that she'd gotten drunk the night before she fell. Did that make her less steady on her feet twelve hours later while changing the light bulb? In earlier conversations, she had admitted to drinking too much alcohol to reduce job stress, which in turn was amplified by the anxiety of self-doubt. She said the drinking helped her relax and feel more confident.

What, then, do we treat: the wrist, the alcohol use, the sensations of anxiety, or the self-doubt? An integrative approach would treat all of it. I spend a good deal of time with patients on this foreign idea that we must look at the whole of their lives. With every symptom, whether a back pain or a headache, it's worth tracing the lines from the particular to the Whole, to map the big picture of what's occurring in mind, body, and spirit.

It helps to remember this when we're exposed to ads and commercials for health products or medications or alternative therapies offering quick, easy fixes. While some of them may be helpful, reaching the pinnacles of wellbeing almost always takes more than one ingredient or product.

Criticism of holism

Critics of holism have accused it of being a *deus ex machina*, which originally referred to a plot device in ancient Greek drama in which a dilemma created by humans was solved by a god in the unlikely nick of time. To the audience, it seemed arbitrary, as the protagonists hadn't relied on their own ingenuity or courage for the solution. Since then, *deus ex machina* has come to mean an artificial solution. In the eyes of some scientists, this is a problem with holism. Attributing clinical outcomes to an intangible like the Whole is, in their eyes, slipshod thinking. Some scientists believe that with the mapping of the entire human genome, a full accounting of the mechanisms of disease and health will be available, putting to rest the rumblings of holism. But since so many philosophers, saints, and scientists have advocated an integral, holistic view of the universe throughout the centuries, that seems unlikely.

An appreciation for the power of the Whole comes easier to the mind that is intuitive. This respect was strong in the ancients, who knew intimately the flesh of earth and the breath of sky, who grasped the wisdom in green creeks and red rock, sandy desert and cobalt sky, the choral harmony in the birth of birds, wolves, foals. Seeing the stamp of wisdom engraved everywhere in the visible world, they revered nature and bowed to its erudition.

Along similar lines, Arthur Rimbaud, the young and troubled French poet, wrote in the nineteenth century that the poet's task was to steal fire from heaven, from the realm of the Unknown. This theft, he said in his earlier years, came from disordering the senses and destroying our habitual way of seeing things. Poetry's purpose was to uncover the divine that had gotten obscured by our half-hearted, superficial glances at the world. Similar intentions drove Prometheus to steal fire from Mount Olympus to bring the gods' magic to humankind

The practicalities

Our next step, then, is to think of the practical applications of an idea as broad and diffuse as the Whole. Fortunately, this idea is highly applicable, and the following is a sequence of thought for seeing both our health and illnesses in its light.

First: when a symptom occurs, remember that it's a message and not a problem. The symptom may be uncomfortable, painful, or even agonizing, but it's not a problem. Instead, it's precisely that which points to the problem. It's your personal assistant, at your service, guiding you toward diagnosis and treatment. In the long run, it's taking you by the shoulders and turning you toward a life which will have you more inclined to whistle or hum in the shower.

Second: trace a path back from the symptom to the whole, and inquire into what it's saying about your life and your body overall. What's the message here? On occasion, it's obvious, but more often than not, it's baffling. This may require some sleuthing, being as observant of details and patterns as Hercule Poirot or Sherlock Holmes. With a close look at what happened around the time of the symptom's occurrence and at what makes it better or worse, you may start to see patterns. It also helps to notice your emotions when the symptom wakens from its slumber. Angry, resigned, depressed, anxious? The feelings and moods that seem to be the result of the symptom may in fact be contributing to the symptom's persistence.

Look at the big picture, the Whole, beyond the symptoms and its dynamics, even if it seems unrelated to the immediate discomfort. Are you eating well, resting, and exercising enough? What needs to change in your life? Which vitamins and minerals are missing? How unhappy are you, and with what? Are you living with integrity? Are you acting in accord with your values and your purpose? Do you have purpose?

In searching for the roots of the symptom, we can go short to the part that hurts or go long to the Whole. Whether we're dealing with a muscle sprain or heart disease, it all makes more sense in light of the Whole. Many back pains, for example, occur in a house of tears and anguish that will never show on an X-ray. So a good habit to acquire is to think "Whole" any time a symptom occurs.

As an example, if you get colds often, the pattern of frequency is itself a message. Each cold is not an isolated event, but a report card on your terrain. Instead of fighting only its symptoms, you can look at your diet, exercise, stress levels, sleep, overall wellbeing, and then see if herbs, supplements, exercise, and catalytic treatments might help rebuild your immune system from the ground up. If the terrain is a toxic mess, then fixing one spot—the symptom—may have little impact. Removing a cancerous tumor is one thing. But profoundly improving the whole biochemical terrain out which the cancer grew is another thing entirely, and an essential treatment strategy in integrative medicine.

If, on the other hand, the terrain is lush and fertile, then that cold or that painful knee will improve faster. It helps to re-educate yourself to look past the specific incident and discover what change it's asking of you on the larger scale. This is crucial because *sometimes the answer lies only in the Whole*. Without taking the terrain into account, treating a symptom can be like spraying foam on an electrical fire instead of turning off the power. So the solution, in these cases, is not to be found in any proximate causes but in invigorating all of mind and body. Unfortunately, to our society, this is a counterintuitive view.

I belabor this point because patients always ask me questions about the body part that hurts, and I usually redirect the conversation to the Whole containing that part. If the flames of a headache are being fanned by eating poorly, overworking, feeling powerless and resentful at home, how can herbs, acupuncture, or pills from the pharmacy be sufficient?

For some people, the commute may be a grind, the job a bore, the marriage a quiet hell. It's precisely this sort of squalid terrain that becomes the breeding ground for illness. In one well-designed study of about 30,000 men and women in fifty-two countries, researchers found that the increased risk of having a heart attack from emotional stress was only slightly less than that of a lifetime of smoking cigarettes. Of the nine identified risk factors for a heart attack, emotional stress was third—a greater risk than high blood pressure, diabetes, and obesity. This is a remarkable finding given the scientific view that focuses primarily on the physical elements of disease.

When the ache or creak comes, any health assessment that doesn't account for the terrain may miss the diagnosis. For some physical ailments, loneliness and estrangement are the real diagnoses and love is the cure. If powerlessness and frustration are the diagnoses, audacity is the cure. When the Whole is intact, we're graced with both a lightness of being and a hardiness that can't be defined by any single measure such as blood pressure or estrogen levels. This vibrant core of healing is the ballroom dance between love, power, beauty, and soul. To paraphrase Emily Dickinson, it can dazzle you slowly.

Personally responsible

This broader perspective easily segues into the idea that we are each responsible for our health. While we've often heard this, it hasn't made a substantial difference in our culture or in the healthcare system yet. For the most part, we still expect health professionals to pick up the pieces of our broken lifestyles. The good news is that taking responsibility for your health contains a hopeful message: it restores you, the patient, and not some external authority, to the pivotal center of your health concerns. In the most hopeful of meta-messages, it says that you are influential, you do have power, you wield lightning bolts.

Your lifestyle choices and your health are two faces of the same coin. Remembering this will make you less likely to think of the body as a valet, or to indulge your proclivity to bend, fold, and irritate it in the service of your personal or professional aspirations. With the frenetic pressures of life in the twenty-first century, the body has become a tool, not a temple. When our lifestyle choices lead to pain and illness, we think nothing of asking someone else to fix it for us. No one's to blame for this logic, as there's no training in our schools or in our culture to teach us otherwise. But now is a good time, early in the twenty-first century, for a fresh new look.

Unless Jason had dedicated himself to remodeling his entire life, I doubt that any therapies, whether medications, surgery, or individual holistic therapies, would have helped keep his former symptoms at bay. The healer in this case was Jason himself, dealing with the diagnosis of lifestyle toxicity. His life as a whole, not any isolated part of it, was a pain factory. No one else—not the smartest team of health professionals in the world—could have done what he did for himself. He was the chief executive savior of his own life.

The idea that we are responsible for our health is not a judgment or a moral assessment. Responsibility in this sense refers to ownership: regardless of the source of the symptoms, even if that source is criminal aggression by another, I am the owner of my health, my pain, my wellness. It happens here in my body, and therefore, it's mine. As Fritz Perls used to say, we are response-able.

Of course, a health professional is, in many cases, the only appropriate person to consult. But that's a different subject. At times, the disease must be treated directly through medications and surgery. I've had some patients with certain conditions who came in adamant that I should treat them because they believe in holism, in my natural healing methods, and hate surgery and medications. In some of those cases, I've almost had to shove them out the door, equally adamant that they must see a medical doctor because I believed that surgery or medications were the only solutions.

But if the disordered terrain must be corrected first, multiple surgeries or medications may be of limited use, even harmful. The whimsy of fate and the blueprint of genetics can lead to illnesses beyond our control. Serious, complex diseases are not amenable to self-diagnosis or self-treatment. But even with serious illnesses, whether it's breast cancer or multiple sclerosis, we can cultivate a lush, fertile terrain with diet, exercise, relaxation, and a soul at peace. Experts can guide us with their skills, while we take responsibility for our role in gardening the terrain.

Enabling in the helping professions

A quick side tour into the principles of addictions treatment may help to better illustrate this idea of responsibility. Experienced members of twelve-step programs such as Alcoholics Anonymous and Narcotics Anonymous counsel newcomers about the perils of enabling—the unintended worsening of an addiction through our good intentions. Out of kindness and the desire to help, friends and family often protect an addict from the consequences of her behavior by making excuses to the boss, by picking up the slack for family responsibilities, or by inaction such as suffering in silence when setting firm limits would be better. All these actions, while well intentioned, can feed the addiction by buffering its painful effects for the addict.

The experts in addictions treatment generally agree that hitting bottom is a turning point, and sometimes, the only solution. Letting the addict feel the body blows of drinking or drugging is, paradoxically, therapeutic in the end. This might include, for example, the spouse declaring the intention to leave the marriage unless the drinking or drugging stops. This sort of dis-enabling, so to speak, is no simple task, as the risk of serious harm or death is always on the horizon if an addict is left entirely on her own to deal with the consequences. This understandably makes friends and family queasy. But enabling is found elsewhere too, such as in parenting, where protecting our children from every hard knock weakens them.

A similar enabling can also occur, in more subtle ways, in the relationship between a patient and health professional. If a doctor of any type of medicine focuses on only eliminating the symptom, the source may be neglected: the patient's lifestyle choices and the value system behind them. Ignoring the symptom's context, or the Whole, sends two meta-messages to the patient: first, that the broken window is the problem; second, the professional will be the one to fix it. Health professionals, out of compassion, professionalism, and altruism, can become unwitting enablers. I'll attest to how the irresistible desire to do good often overrides sensible judgment. Ultimately, a health professional's job should be to assist patients in acquiring the horsepower to generate health on their own. While there are places like the emergency room where the only job is to pull the patient off the edge of a cliff, the work in most clinics could use less enabling.

A large part of the work in integrative medicine is focused on the patient's lifestyle and emotions. This is the Whole, the womb of either optimal vitality or illness, for the flourishing or the deterioration of the human body and spirit. Attending to Jason's leg and hip pain alone would have been to miss the mark. Without knowing that his lifestyle itself was the real problem, we might have delayed his transformation. The knowledge he has gained, and the skills he has learned for creating a balanced lifestyle, will now support him for the rest of his life.

In the point-blank, here-and-now, everyday encounters with the fervors of the human body, we are faced with a naked choice: we are making ourselves either healthier or less so. Sitting on the couch is not nothing: it is a something that worsens health—not detectably, not much, but it's nevertheless a dose of inertia, an act of stillness. It's an act because it affects the body. Unlike a mechanical object where no wear equals no tear, the human body deteriorates without motion. With regard to nutrition, eating pretzels and potato chips on the weekend won't put you in the hospital, but the cumulative effects of eating pseudofoods over a lifetime are potentially dangerous. So we are pressed skin-to-skin against the perpetual, Heraclitean motion of the human body moving ever so slightly, one nanosecond to the next, in one direction or another, between better and worse, between ascent and descent. We either proactively create a healthy life, or we slip downhill a step at a time—perhaps slowly and undetectably—by the smallest of measures.

Samuel Taylor Coleridge, of *The Rime of the Ancient Mariner* fame, wrote philosophically about the relationship of the part to the Whole:

> *A symbol is characterized by a translucence of the special in the particular,*
> *or of the general in the special, or the universal in the general:*
> *above all by the translucence of the eternal through and in the temporal.*

Coleridge echoes the opinions of other thinkers we've met so far when he says that the particular, which for us might be a hip or knee, is a symbol of the universal and the eternal. We're always connected, everywhere we go and in every manner conceivable, to the Whole.

In a similar vein, one thousand five-hundred years before Coleridge, Greek philosopher Plotinus wrote:

> *Beauty is the translucence, through the material phenomenon,*
> *of the eternal splendor of the One.*

Remembering the Whole can remind us of the healing promise churning in the wellspring of the body and in all of nature. It can remind us that the human body is an allusion of deeper truths, a logo of spiritual possibility, one fleshy, familiar shape of stardust and starlight. The Whole includes not just all of mind and body, and not just our relationship with society and friends, but our intimacy with the cosmos itself as it stretches toward time and space and spirit unimaginable. To think holistically is to explore these outer reaches of human thought and possibility. With that, medicine is no longer just about the physical body. It's an endeavor belonging to the core task of finding and expressing our very human destiny.

A Beautiful Medicine

Chapter Nine

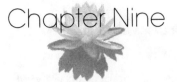

Awake, Aware, Alive

A New Yorker cartoon from some years ago shows a penguin flying above the rest of his huddle. As the other penguins stand on the ice looking up at him, he flaps his wings eagerly and shouts, "Look, we haven't been flapping hard enough!" Today, it's no longer news that beliefs and expectations shape our lives, for better or for worse. The cartoon reminds us to innovate, to pulverize fossilized beliefs, to unearth treasures of the unexpected, to consider better ways of commuting between icebergs.

The relevance of this to medicine is that the real diagnosis hidden behind the diagnostic codes we submit to insurance companies is, in many cases, what Albert Einstein called optical illusion. When, as he wrote, breaking free of this illusion leads to greater affection, to being unrestricted to our personal desires, and to compassion for all living creatures, then we can better inhale the air of human possibility.

A glad heart is good for the body. And conversely, when the heart is troubled, the body becomes a forum of protest. The universe within us impresses itself on the body through pace, posture, shape, and physiology. In particular, our beliefs, including our self-esteem and our outlooks gloomy or bright, are the silhouettes of our choices. They in turn mold the contours of our health. Our beliefs about ourselves and others are, at best, slightly misshapen symbols of reality, and at worst, caricatures. Any warping and buckling of our perceptions—one of the most common being the belief that

A human being is part of the whole that we call the universe, a part limited in time and space. He experiences himself, his thoughts and feelings, as something separated from the rest—a kind of optical illusion of his consciousness. This illusion is a prison for us, restricting us to our personal desires and to affection for only the few people nearest us. Our task must be to free ourselves from this prison by widening our circle of compassion to embrace all living beings and all of nature.

–Albert Einstein

we're inadequate or inferior—adds to the junkyard of our discontent. Einstein paralleled the sayings of mystics when he suggested that being free of these distorting beliefs will help us be more compassionate. It often requires us to flap harder, or at least to see that we've been stuck in assumptions about what flapping can do.

To begin our inquiry into this idea, here's more about Karen, with the angry alcoholic father, whom we met in Chapter Two.

Karen's assumptions

As if Karen didn't have enough tensions in her life, she had another conflict troubling her. Her three brothers were angry because they believed, mistakenly, that she had stolen money from their mother as she was dying in a nursing home some years ago. Although Karen had used the money to pay for medical care and the nursing home, the brothers were unconvinced. As a result, she became estranged from all three brothers after their mother died.

More recently, she'd been increasingly anxious about an upcoming family reunion. As the date approached, she noticed how her anxiety aggravated her pain. I suggested to Karen that she pay close attention to the way her stress triggered her pain, as it could provide useful information.

One day, we discussed Buber's idea that "every loving deed is a true deed," as well as the similar "every loving thought is true and everything else is an appeal for help and healing" from *A Course in Miracles*. If she were to think of her brothers' anger in this light, then their anger wasn't "true." She could see it as unintentional pretense, obscuring their love for her, and choose to see that their anger wasn't the final and defining measure of their relationship to her. She could hypothesize that they loved her, that their behavior eclipsed a kinder truth. While the brothers might be unaware of their love for her, convinced otherwise by their own anger, Karen could still test the hypothesis and see how they responded.

Feeling nervous but determined, she went to the family reunion. This estrangement had disturbed the extended family, so all eyes would be on her and the brothers. After walking into the reception area at the restaurant, she went straight to one of the brothers, took his face in her hands, kissed him, and said, "It's great

> There are more things in heaven and earth, Horatio, than are dreamt of in your philosophy.
>
> –William Shakespeare

to see you again." His face softened, and he warmed up to her instantly. In a second, years of resentment vanished in the breeze. After she greeted her other two brothers similarly, they too warmed up in seconds. With years of tension disappearing in moments, Karen was elated, though slightly stunned at her own power. Once she saw the leverage she had, she better understood how our worlds are shaped by assumptions.

After coming home, she noticed that her physical pain came less often. It became clearer to her that although a physical trauma had started the pain, anxiety aroused it. For months afterward, she was pain-free for longer periods of time, and she reported "feeling great." The only aggravations of the pain came from the occasional stresses of daily living. Once Karen understood her own fear underlying her assumptions about the brothers, and considered other possible explanations for their behavior, she broke through the impasse that appeared to have been of their doing. When she could remember her pain was communication, a message, it was no longer a problem but an ally on her path to transformation. It reminded her to relax, to care, to love.

We are subjective people living in our subjective worlds. What seems real is often just projection, an unconscious fabrication of our worst fears played out on a movie screen between us and the world. The psychologist, saint, and philosopher have long accepted the garbled influence of projection as a given of the human condition. If we remember this, we can consciously design our own lens through which we see the world—easier said than done, but possible.

As we explore the limitations and the malleability of perception, a quick tour of a few provocative and puzzling ideas in science may help. I'll start with a few that remind us of how little we see.

Biological blinders

We know from the most basic biology that our senses take in far less than those of most animals. If we had the eyes of an American kestrel falcon, we'd be able to see an insect about the size of a pinhead from nearly sixty feet in the air. If we had the nose of a dog, we'd be able to smell epileptic seizures before they happened and substances buried forty feet underground. A dog's sense of smell is a hundred thousand times better than is ours. If we had the sonar of a bat, we'd be able to distinguish between a mosquito and a gnat in the blackness of night while zipping around at twenty miles an hour, and some of us could detect the sound of a beetle walking. If we had the "nose" of one type of moth, we'd be able to pick up the scent of the pheromones of other moths seven miles away. That's over 36,000 feet, the altitude at which many jet airliners fly. While the human ear can pick up sounds ranging from 20 to 20,000 hertz, the latter being the faintest ping we can hear, a dolphin can hear sounds of up to 150,000 hertz.

Then there's the sea of electromagnetic waves surrounding our bodies at every moment: television programs, cell phone conversations, radio shows, Wi-Fi highways. A kaleidoscope of information by the trillions of bits goes through our flesh without our slightest awareness—a circus of which we're oblivious until we turn on a computer, radio, TV, or cell phone.

Remembering how little we can see, hear, smell, feel, and taste is a good reminder that there are more things in heaven and earth by ratio than are dreamt of in our philosophy.

The four percent

All the above is intriguing, but familiar and believable. Quantum physics, on the other hand, gives us ideas not only bizarre but beyond baffling. While they contort logic and common sense into a pretzel, they're mathematically validated, rigorously tested notions often leading to Nobel Prizes. They just happen to brazenly defy the logic of the world as we know it. Despite their august history and age—some of these ideas have been around for almost a century—they don't much influence the other sciences or the world at large. Maybe it's because their implications are preposterous, strange enough to humble even the wildest fantasy or childhood illusion. Only a few such ideas will be mentioned here.

First, in the 1970s, physicists realized that contrary to previous assumptions, gravity couldn't be the only force holding galaxies together. Instead, their mathematical gymnastics indicated that something mysterious and powerful prevented stars from scattering beyond their galactic orbits into the wilds of outer space. In the 1990s, the answer was found in the discovery of dark matter—a potent, invisible mass that kept galaxies intact. Its effect was similar to that of a magnet in keeping the stars from scattering about. But the baffling part was that dark matter is physical mass we can't see. Imagine telling a friend that you have an invisible rock in your hand.

Then, physicists realized that the concept of dark matter couldn't answer another puzzling question: why was the universe expanding at accelerating speeds? While they knew that galaxies are moving out and away, the reason for this happening at increasingly faster rates was unknown. Physicists then found evidence for *dark energy*, again mass that can't be seen but shapes the motion of all the galaxies in the universe. That helped explain the accelerating speed.

Both dark matter and dark energy have physical mass, just like mountains and moons, but are invisible. Physicists estimate that dark matter makes up about 23 percent of the physical universe and dark energy about 73 percent. This means that the trillions of stars, planets, and the entire physical universe of which the Earth is a trillionth of a pinpoint is about 4 percent of what's visible. When we look at the space photos of the fragile, blue-green planet we call home, or at the silver moon and gleaming stars, we see 4 percent of what's physically present.

Then we have the yards-long math equations giving us proof on paper for the existence of parallel universes. This idea suggests that there are whole universes like ours that we can't detect yet. We don't have experimental evidence for this, but, after decades of effort, physicists have done the math— and it works.

We also have Bell's theorem, experimentally validated in 1982, showing how one subatomic particle can affect another without any physical connection between them. So, in the most rigorous of sciences, it's been proved, both experimentally and mathematically, that one thing can affect another, at a distance, with no physical connection between them. The name for this is *nonlocality*, an idea first thought of by Einstein and which he called a "spooky distance." Today, it's a given in quantum physics.

In a different but reminiscent light, ancient shamans, priests of the oracle, temple gurus, philosophers of east and west, poets, painters, monks, and nuns have also pursued the mysteries beyond our senses. As though a homing device were sewn into our physical and spiritual DNA, this search has always lured us in efforts fueled by the suspicion that the visible world holds forth illusions. Whether we're searching for a parallel universe through math equations, nirvana through meditation, or heaven through prayer, the charismatic tug of the mysteries is a constant.

Remembering that our senses detect only a fraction of what exists may help in softening the sharp, brittle, mechanistic world constructed by the contemporary mind. As we consider all we don't know, and what we don't know we don't know, we could ask if it's possible that in medicine we can measure only 4 percent of what we need to know about healing. Our beliefs and assumptions are cartoon sketches of reality that give us approximations colored by our fears and longings. Philosophically, we're not flapping our wings hard enough.

The next step then is to explore the relevance of these ideas to an integrative view of health and medicine.

Beliefs, assumptions, and health

Psychology and philosophy both tell us that we live in a world shaped by our assumptions at best and our delusions at worst. On the streets of culture, it's no longer news that the stories of our past, including the imprimatur of our childhoods, influence our present and future lives. That we can be fooled by our senses is generally well understood in basic psychology, psychotherapy, and self-help programs.

I will footnote, however, that the powerful results of changing beliefs, such as those we saw in Karen's life, do not necessarily equate with the popular saying "You create your own reality," which is a good idea on steroids. That a bias can distort perception is well documented. Few of us would question the effect of self-fulfilling prophecies, of expectations influencing results. The placebo effect, that sentry dog of medical research, remains largely unquestioned.

But to say that we create reality implies that everything is relative and that all personal reality is invented. This goes to a philosophical extreme in a subject that our brightest philosophers have been unable to resolve after grappling with it for centuries. Among other difficulties, it implies a complete moral and philosophical relativism. That would put us on shaky conceptual footing. I once heard a seminar leader say that because we're making it all up in language and we're creating our own realities, there is no good or bad, no right or wrong.

I suspect that the idea of creating your own reality is easy to assume after seeing people's lives change dramatically from dismantling their misperceptions. Had Karen been creating her own reality and had she created another? At first, it would seem so. As idiom, it works fine. But it's an imprecise way of speaking about something more complex than it first appears to be. That a technique is powerful doesn't mean it's the primary and entire measure of human inquiry. Creating your own reality is a great idea with holes, as the absence of an objective reality is a hard theoretical pill to swallow. Few philosophers have gone that far. The Advaita Vedanta tradition in Hinduism, along with other traditions, says that everything exists only in the eyes of God, Brahman, or Consciousness, but it also blends this idea with a moral absolutism. Good and bad, right and wrong, are embedded, they say, in the inherent design of the universe, an idea echoed in Christianity, Judaism, Buddhism, and all the major religions of the world.

Another approach would be to think that although an objective reality does exist, we can only know it through our biases. We can only know our personal versions of the world, colored by our fear and longing, our loves and aversions. In this view, we don't create reality but whittle and sculpt it to bring forth transformative changes. For thousands of years, we've heard of this in stories ranging from Plato's cave shadows to the Native American coyote as trickster to *The Matrix* from Hollywood.

Epistemology, the study of how we know what we know, and how to break free of our illusions, has been of perpetual interest for thinkers from Plato to Hans-Georg Gadamer, from Kant and Nietzsche to Gregory Bateson, from the *maya* of Hinduism to the *avijja* of Buddhism, from Gestalt theory to cognitive therapy. Sage and pundit agree that "seeing the world as it is" is a confounding, if not impossible, task.

Chilean neurobiologists Francisco Varela and Humberto Maturana wrote in their book *The Tree of Knowledge* about their lab experiments with frogs' vision that strongly suggested that we can't know the world as it is.

After the frogs' eyes were surgically altered to look 180 degrees in a different direction, the frogs' aim with their tongues didn't adjust accordingly as they sought prey. They kept missing their prey by exactly 180 degrees, though common sense would tell us that they—and we, if likewise altered— would simply move our bodies to compensate for the change.

Maturana and Varela concluded that we don't perceive the world, but instead, we only know the impressions that the world makes on our senses. It's as though we're inside a large balloon seeing the shape of hands pressing in. In other words, they say, all human experience is an internal event. When someone touches your arm, the warmth and pressure are your internal experience, and you are therefore experiencing yourself. Although your experience of yourself has been changed by the other person, it's all happening inside you—you're feeling sensations in your brain triggered by a change in the nerve endings in your skin. There is someone out there, but we can only know our internal experience of that person.

The epistemological precision of this idea was captured in a bumper sticker of some years ago that read, "Just because I'm paranoid, it doesn't mean they're not out to get me."

The ancient wisdom traditions have been especially insistent, each in its own way, that our normal states of mind occur in a sort of dream world. That may seem far-fetched, as the world seems solid and appears to work fairly consistently. But it's not as fanciful as it sounds. The reach of animal senses and the discoveries in physics that we've examined remind us of the blinders we wear. But theory aside, the challenge is first to actually see our biases and the way they shape the selectivity of our eyes, and then to change them. Just as the eye can't see itself because it's doing the looking, so our biases can't see themselves—a bias is the very instrument with which we make sense of things. But we rarely feel biased, and there's the rub.

How is all this relevant to health? The degree to which we are awake and aware affects the body. Beliefs and biases, and the ensuing moods and emotions, can change blood chemistry, including brain chemistry. If I'm convinced that I am unloved and am perennially facing the danger of social rejection, then my brain, my adrenal glands, my heart, my immune system, and more will upset the chemistry in my body. Our moods depend a good deal on our perceptions and assumptions about ourselves and others, and therefore, they directly and instantly change our physiology.

Behind that, our values, beliefs, and aspirations shape the architecture of our lifestyles, including the pace of our lives, choice of careers, attitudes about living, care of the body. They in turn affect the flow and quality of blood in our veins. They can even shape the body, as witnessed by a person becoming permanently slouched in discouragement or made tall and straight with confidence.

Here, the story of the broken window can once again help. As we trace the roots of a symptom into the past, we find a long family history shaped by values, priorities, and choices that lead eventually to the broken window. The roadways of the family's values and belief systems shape the traffic of their words, actions, and lifestyle, which in turn affect the physiology of the body. If lifestyle habits insult the body, they can drain our adrenal glands, raise our blood sugar, strain our cardiovascular systems, dent our immune systems, and injure any system in the body. A chronic symptom is often the tail end of years of unhealthy food, inadequate sleep, minimal exercise, too much stress, a pressured lifestyle, and not enough love. In many chronic diseases, this is the core of the matter, and therefore crucial in understanding the etiology of the patient's condition.

A dilemma for the health professional is that treating only the symptom may inadvertently enable a patient to continue grinding her life force down to a nub. In using clinical tools, we do best when addressing the core of the issue, not the broken window, and when we are patient and persistent in learning how the baseball bat got to the scene of the crime. Julie's story was a clear example of this. She had gotten into the habit of using the calming and energizing effects of acupuncture to blunt the distress of her too-long work weeks, junk food diet, and a six-pack or two of beer every night. Once she and I reached the understanding that I'd been enabling her, she changed her life as only she could, a task beyond the reach of any health professional.

In many medical cases, to use Einstein's terms, the true diagnosis is optical illusion, and the treatment illumination. The illusion of being unloved and other such fancies can rattle the nerves, depress blood chemistry, and twist the spine into knots. In contrast, finding the warm, clear places of serenity and caring in the heart can help flood the body with the waters of vitality and healing.

As we continue to look at the role of belief and assumptions in healing, a quick look at the placebo effect may help.

Harnessing the placebo effect: real magic

If a drug performs no better than a placebo in a research study, then that drug is considered ineffective. All medical researchers know a new drug must outperform placebo—the proverbial, inert "sugar pill"—if the study is to meet the highest standards in the field. In this context, the placebo's only job is to be the spoiler that points to a weakness in the contender. It's an idea largely unquestioned in the world of medical research.

But this means that every medical researcher believes in the mind's ability to improve the body. This is a curious blind spot in the conventional scientific view, when the extraordinary power of belief and assumption to heal the body should be celebrated in a scientific Mardi Gras. Instead, this power continues to be seen through a keyhole: it's respected, with the title of placebo, only as a tool in the kit box for weeding out impostors. In contrast, the psyche's influence on the body is celebrated in integrative medicine, where it is intentionally harnessed to support health and healing.

Hypnosis is one example of the power of belief, assumption, and subconscious programming in healing the body. In 1995, the National Institutes of Health issued a report on the best and latest research on the subject. It stated that sufficient evidence exists for the effectiveness of mind-body techniques such as hypnosis and relaxation methods. In a strong endorsement, NIH stated that there is sufficient evidence for the effect of hypnosis on cancer pain, and in chronic pain conditions including irritable bowel syndrome, oral mucositis, temporomandibular disorders, and tension headaches. All this from belief, assumption, and expectation planted intentionally in the patient's mind.

Beliefs, assumptions, expectations, suppositions—all these can affect our physical health to varying degrees in myriad ways. To repeat, these are often the true diagnoses hiding behind the ones with numbered codes that we send to the insurance companies and Medicare. To reduce any possible confusion, I must note again that many cases of disease are purely physical in origin, unrelated to belief or expectation. This includes childhood cancers, pathogen-induced diseases, poverty-induced malnutrition, or congenital diseases, among many more.

Expectations and medicine

If beliefs and assumptions are at times the core diagnosis, they're an essential part of any medical framework for diagnosis. If a person believes she'll get better, then according to the ways of placebo, this will improve the chances she'll recover. In addition, if the angst of unresolved grief, anger, or terror is feeding the physical pain, attempts to treat only the physical symptoms may lead to frustration.

Assumptions can cramp possibility. With the expectation that a medical condition is permanent or intractable, whether it's because a patient thinks she's too old or that there's no cure, the expectation itself will influence the results. We might decide to leave a few stones unturned or to proceed half-hearted. For many diseases, the odds of healing really are slim to zero. But while it's unethical for a health professional to promise a cure, it also helps to avoid convincing the patient that healing is impossible except in the most obvious circumstances. This won't guarantee any results, but when a patient is receptive to unforeseen possibilities, the odds for healing are improved. She may flap her wings harder. Why not stay in an attitude of possibility and unfettered receptivity to the unexpected? As we might have expected, the illness may in fact worsen. But how adamant and convinced should we be that we won't heal in a world where we can only see 4 percent of what's there?

Many illnesses considered permanent or incurable have vanished, either spontaneously or as the result of clinical efforts. The story of Ann, who at eighty-six saw stage IV lung cancer disappear, is a good reminder to keep our arms open to the unpredictable, the unexpected, and the remarkable. Since this is only one anecdote, it doesn't hold much sway in the world of medical research. But with millions of anecdotes spanning five thousand years all over the planet, it should at least provoke our curiosity—that essential characteristic of scientific inquiry—and open the gates of discovery a bit wider.

Another common myth, as we have seen, is that aging causes disease. As we have seen, *chronological aging does not cause disease*. It vastly increases the odds of disease, and at the very end, the result of aging is obvious and inevitable. But strictly speaking, it is not "the cause" of many of old age's infirmities. To condense a long story, it's more accurate to say aging greatly increases our susceptibility to disease. An undeniable correlation exists between aging and the onset of aches, pains, and disease. But increased susceptibility to disease from aging is not the same as the direct cause of a disease.

The logic usually goes like this: I'm getting older, my symptoms are caused by aging, and since I can't get younger, this problem is going to get worse. That's acceptable logic, but the premises are inaccurate. It's been shown repeatedly that if we halt or reverse the biological aging that results from neglect or misuse of the body, then we improve the chances of healing. As we saw in Chapter Three, The Wellspring of Healing, oxidation, or the "rusting" of the body, increases with age but is often reversible. Here's one story to illustrate what can happen as we get older.

Rachel was in her late seventies when she came to see me while recovering from a mastectomy and chemotherapy for breast cancer. Feeling exhausted and lifeless from the chemotherapy, she wanted help in feeling better. She'd been retired for many years, and gave me the impression, as do many retirees, that the model for retirement as a time to relax, do little, or do only what we want, wasn't working for her. She also believed that she was on the decline—a reasonable conclusion as she approached her eighties in a country where she'd already exceeded the average life span of a woman born in the 1930s. As I listened to her during the early months of our work together, I heard nothing in her words that implied a future for her. In fact, she hinted several times that she might be at the beginning of the end. A perception of that sort is not just a neutral observation—it actively shapes our decisions, and therefore our physical health.

Over the next three years, we worked together; she came often for acupuncture and we talked at length about her life. We discussed a conflict with loved ones, which she eventually resolved. She took vitamin D3, multivitamins, and electrolyte solutions for boosting cellular vitality. She ate more whole foods and exercised more. Early on, she saw the merits of becoming more engaged with her world. We discussed her retirement as an opportunity to engage meaningfully with her community, so she started to contribute more by teaching, mentoring, and volunteering. Over a three-year span, she went from a dearth of activity to being overscheduled at times.

As a result of her renewed involvement with work, her self-esteem improved. She developed a fresh vision for her life. When her good deeds were mirrored back to her through having her photo and press releases in the local media, she was inspired. She recognized that the stresses of work or volunteering were opportunities to grow, not something to retire from at any age. Eventually, as her life took on a different complexion, she became far more animated. You could see the aliveness, the *élan vital*, in her face, body, and arms as she spoke. This is what happened between the ages of seventy-seven and eighty: three years of aging had seen a reversal of a decline. She was more vibrant, alive, and cheerful at eighty than she had been at seventy-seven. This is what can happen as we age.

Virginia, at the age of seventy-nine, came to me for fatigue and overall malaise. As she began to improve with acupuncture, she noticed that her moods were also improving, but best of all, so were her artistic inspiration and the quality of her art. Then during the second winter after starting treatments, she developed a troubling cardiac arrhythmia. During this time, she seemed frail, and I was concerned. But with a combination of acupuncture, nutritional supplements, and medication adjustments from her cardiologist, the arrhythmia disappeared. Eventually, she stabilized and all was well. She felt better than she had in years. After aging a couple of years, between the ages of seventy-nine and eighty, her life went from cloudy to bright.

The belief that suffering is inevitable after we reach fifty or sixty is rampant in our society. Sure, aches and pains seem to find us quicker and more often than before. We can't hold off the pain and deterioration forever. But more possibility is available than we're inclined to think. While no one can promise miracles, and we know that death waits for all of us at the end of the corridor, it helps to cast off the belief that the calendar is the cause of pain and suffering in our later years. Misuse, underuse, neglect, oxidation, cell degeneration, dehydration—yes. But not calendar aging as the direct causal agent of pain and disease.

Today, seventy is looking younger than ever before. We've all seen fit, healthy, vibrant people in their eighties who are in better shape than are others in their fifties. When rock stars like Mick Jagger and Paul McCartney shout and prance about on stage at ages far past the minimum eligibility for AARP membership, and when Helen Klein runs monthly marathons at eighty-four, we need to redefine aging.

The span between fifty and eighty is chronologically the same number of years between twenty and fifty. For some reason, the former sounds shorter. But during our later years, we still have ample time to encourage the body to regenerate. We can be productive, learn new skills, grow muscles, flex better, run faster, laugh bigger. It's all possible, but only if we're willing to do what nourishes and strengthens soul, mind, and body. That's the challenge: *the price of admission includes exercise, discipline in eating well, making the time for self-care, and being at peace with yourself and the people in your life. It doesn't come free.*

Taking care of our health through ample exercise, excellent food, and a happy heart increases the odds of dancing until the lights go out. But the requirements for health have been redesigned in the last thirty years. As I mentioned earlier, the devotion to exercise and healthy foods that would have made your neighbors gawk in 1970 is today's ideal.

Healing in layers: becoming conscious

As we return to the relationship between seeing, understanding, and healing, which we discussed in light of the connection between consciousness and health, another element of healing is worth noting.

Healing often happens in layers, like peeling off layers of clothing we've worn on a cold day. We've already seen this in the stories of Linda, Joan, Alma, Cheryl, and others, where the disappearance of physical symptoms led to an emotional discharge. The reverse can occur as well, where an emotional resolution or release can lead to the disappearance of a physical pain. To expand on the idea a little further, it helps to know that aside from our simple and occasional ailments, our more complex or chronic symptoms may improve in layers, like the layers of an onion. These stages or layers can be physical, psychological, or both. To illustrate, here are a few examples.

Doreen came in for her second treatment and reported that her low back pain had slightly improved. But as the pain improved, a rash had appeared on the inside of her right arm, then vanished after a few hours. When I asked if anything similar had occurred before, she said she'd had poison oak in that exact spot three years earlier. In the following week, she came for her third visit and reported another slight improvement in her back pain. But a rash like the first had appeared on her other arm, and it too vanished quickly without fanfare. It appeared at the spot where she'd had poison oak five years earlier.

We were peeling layers of unfinished healing, first from three years ago, then from five years ago. It was debris forgotten in the basement, being hauled out in a thorough housecleaning from the bottom up. For some reason, the toxins from the poison oak hadn't been completely flushed from her body before.

Another patient, Betty, was a young nurse whom I hadn't treated for about a year or so. She came in for fatigue and the last tremors of a migraine. The day after her treatment, her head had felt much better and her exhaustion had improved, but she had broken out in a red, oozing rash on her arms, shoulders, and half her torso. Five years earlier, she'd gotten poison ivy at exactly the same places, badly enough that she was admitted to the hospital and put on steroid medications. As with Doreen, this was a cleansing, so it quickly went away.

Both Betty and Doreen went through a detoxification, the elimination of waste, not the birth of new symptoms. The rashes weren't problems, but the last gasping breaths of decontamination at work. Since the cells hadn't flushed away the toxicity of the rashes when they first occurred, they had waited for years until stimulated to finally clean house.

In these and many other cases, the detoxification is just physical. But as we've seen, the idea of detox also applies to the emotional self. When people start to heal, they often encounter the next layers of unfinished work: the remnants of unresolved trauma such as sexual abuse, the death of a child, or the loss of a husband. Like the layers of rock we see where a highway cuts through a mountainside, unresolved stresses can accumulate in layers. They can be either physical, as in the case of Betty and Doreen, or both emotional and physical, as with Linda, Joan, and Alma.

Susan was in her mid-thirties when she came to see me, tired of what seemed like an endless string of sinus infections and chest colds over the years, and looking for a treatment other than the antibiotics she usually received. After starting acupuncture, she quickly started to feel better overall during a course of five or six treatments, barely feeling the sensations of the inserted needles. But then during one visit, a needle I put into her wrist caused an unusually strong pain that led her to sob uncontrollably.

After a few minutes, she recognized this profound sadness as precisely what she'd felt as an eleven-year-old during her parents' ugly divorce. She said she felt as though she were experiencing the grief exactly as it had occurred back then, or perhaps even for the first time. The crying wouldn't stop even after she went home, as though it had a life of its own, and she cried herself to sleep several nights in a row. "It was crazy," she said, referring to the utter surprise of dealing with emotions she thought she'd put away twenty-four years earlier. When her grieving drew to a close after two weeks, her emotional boundaries had broadened to make space for a truth from her past.

Five years later, she told me that the event had been profound and life-changing—not that she felt resolved about the divorce or about the distance that still existed between her and her father—but that the truth was now in full view. The pain in Susan's wrist came from prying open the frozen locks of her grief. None of the previous acupuncture points had hurt at all. Only later did I tell her that the point was on the lung meridian, which in Chinese medicine is connected not only with the lungs but with sorrow. After that experience and the series of treatments five years ago, Susan stopped suffering from colds or sinusitis.

An important but largely unrecognized clinical issue is that the clinician must be able to recognize when a symptom is a detox reaction, the messiness of housecleaning—whether emotional or biological. This sort of reaction is a sign that the body is getting better, however awful it may feel. In these cases, the discomfort shouldn't be suppressed with substitutive methods and attacked as another disease. Instead, it should either be left alone or even encouraged to progress, to go further with its work. If either the body or mind is feeling unwell from the pains of new possibilities being born, then controlling or substitutive methods should be used only if the stress or pain is too much to bear. Otherwise, the health professional is suppressing the very dynamics of healing.

Catalytic methods are best to help things along, just like midwifery, to encourage the passage through rough transitions and to support its further expression. Otherwise, a valuable opportunity for healing will be lost. In the future, when the body or mind tries detoxing again in the same way, the pain and stress may be just as strong, if not stronger.

When we ask if a symptom is real or if it's psychological, we ask a flawed question. The analogies of the Smith Island cake and the broken window, as well as Stanislav Grof's idea of the coex mentioned in Chapter Two, suggest a model in which symptoms are often complex, layered events with different faces. Since the physical and the psychological aspects of human experience blend like sugar and tea, then, to greater or lesser degrees, symptoms include both.

If we say depression is a neurochemical problem, or that a stomach problem *is* all in your head, then we're implying that there is a single cause and that it's either physical or psychological. This *either/or* thinking is misleading, simplistic, and mechanistic. Although sugar and tea blend into one taste, they're different nevertheless. Similarly, a neurochemical dysfunction can't be the whole story behind depression and other psychological challenges. It will always include fears, doubts, anger, loneliness, and other such threatening creatures on the hero's journey.

In some cases, the neurochemical imbalance might be primary, which means the person won't have a fighting chance until the physical imbalances are corrected first. But the idea that depression or other psychological struggle is *caused* by a biochemical deficit is grossly oversimplified, as shown in the analogy of the broken window. When emotional stress triggers a physical symptom, we need to ask why the symptom manifests in different ways. When different people undergo the same stress, one person will have insomnia, another migraines, yet another diarrhea, and so on. If the stress were the *cause* of the symptom, these people would all have the same symptom. Instead, the stress becomes a ventriloquist that speaks through a biological weak link unique to each person.

If, for example, we have a tendency to suffer from stomach problems, or anxiety, or high blood pressure, then those become the vulnerable spots attacked by the armies of emotional stress. Unresolved and chronic fear, resentment, loneliness, grief, anxiety, and the like are opportunistic: they take advantage of the weak links in the chain. Once the stress finds a spot, it will set up headquarters there and start issuing distress signals. Since the symptom's job is to be a spokesperson, the stress wants a spot in the body with a booming voice. Given the clamor and din of our pressured lives, it needs to blare its messages at volumes high enough to compete with all the other noise.

Conversely, if a symptom seems to be caused by stress, it's a disservice to the patient to think that it's purely psychological. Even in those cases where an insight or emotional resolution leads to a complete disappearance of the symptom, there had to have been a break in the fence. The mind's efforts need a breach, a weak link, in the physical body. The words psychosomatic and psychogenic overshoot the subtle and complex relationship between mind and body.

One young patient came to me for the treatment of a severe abdominal pain that her doctors said was permanent. She found great relief from her first session of acupuncture. But the day after her pain vanished, all her lymph nodes became swollen. On the following day, she got angry with a family member and the abdominal pain returned while the swelling in her lymph nodes disappeared. One end of a balloon was being squeezed to make the other end larger—a common occurrence in the early stages of healing.

Her opportunity was to see how her emotional stress spoke through her body and to understand herself better. She had also suffered from severe constipation since childhood, and the accumulated toxins were likely to have been the physical basis for her current symptoms. Her symptoms weren't either physical or mental, but both.

The idea of catharsis in psychology can be applied to the body as well: Doreen's poison oak, Betty's poison ivy, and the young woman's swollen lymph nodes were expressions of what we could call catharsis of the body. The term for the uncomfortable experiences that come from detoxing the body is called a Herxheimer's reaction.

Peeling layers of symptoms can be an essential part of healing. Catharsis in both the mind and the body is often at work as these layers peel away—whether it's opening the sluices of unwept tears in the soul or releasing toxins from the bowels. As we remove each layer to reveal more unfinished business, we do best by embracing them and collaborating with them to help them do their job. They're symptoms after all, which means they're doggedly trying to help us. If we listen to them carefully instead of rushing blindly to get rid of them, we might hear the whispering behind the pain and sorrow, the quiet choirs of wisdom. But if we suppress the urgent, cathartic expression of healing, we stop or delay progress.

Crying, for example, is not a problem. When you lose a loved one, when you've suffered rejection, well, you're supposed to cry. The tears prove you're human. And while that may seem obvious, it can be tough to surrender and open the spigot all the way. Crying is a release, a healing experience. The thrust of our humanness pushes us toward healing, wholeness, integration, and wisdom—yes, all that from our silly tears. If we block the healing river of tears with drugs, medications, sweets, alcohol, denial, male or female machismo, we interrupt the rhythms of heaven and earth. In the throes of our raw, aching losses, weeping is the mandatory next step in the hero's journey and a test of spiritual mettle.

Different shapes of awareness

The path to greater self-awareness can assume many forms. It can range from the release of cellular waste triggered by insights into past trauma to the most soul-wrenching trials of emotional catharsis. Whatever the form—physical, emotional, spiritual—it all points to healing as an element of the transformative journey. Same idea, different angles. As we've seen, becoming more conscious is integral to the path of transformation. A truly integrative approach to medicine includes enhancing consciousness, working to dissolve the lines between the physical and the spiritual, the boundaries between the visible and the invisible. Health includes the mandate to discover, learn, to become more conscious, more sensitive, more awake.

Of course, healing doesn't always happen this way. If a child in Bangladesh gets night blindness from vitamin A deficiency, or one in Tanzania gets malaria from a mosquito, or one in Philadelphia suffers from asthma worsened by mold, the roots lie in biological, political, and economic contexts, not in the child's mind. But for most of us living in developed countries, it's worth seeing if our symptoms are pointing us toward greater self-awareness, actualization, discovery, and integration.

Unseen potential of integrative medicine

An exciting world of possibility lies in an integrative approach to health. In looking at the issue of awareness, I'll present one last, simple idea. It's the lack of awareness about the potential of integrative medicine. Year after year, millions of people throughout the world are healing from CAM (complementary and alternative) therapies. But the potential of these methods is still largely unknown, or thought impossible.

Gary was a retired executive who came to me for the treatment of Bell's palsy. Half his face appeared to have melted like wax exposed to heat. Where his left eyelid, cheek, jaw, and lips drooped, he experienced numbness, lack of control, and uncomfortable tingling. Drinking and eating were awkward, as he could control only half his mouth. During one of his first medical evaluations, Gary's neurologist told him there was no cure for the palsy, so he should get used to living with it for the rest of his life. Gary was also told, after he asked, that acupuncture would not help. But he thought he'd give the unknown a try anyway, since the prospect of living his entire life with half a face was more than depressing. After seven acupuncture treatments, Gary's face was 80 percent improved, the signs of the palsy barely noticeable. The potential of natural healing methods will not be fully known for a long time.

In reviewing some of the ideas I've covered so far—the symptom as a message, the wellsprings of possibility, the inherent healing potential of the body—it's clear that more is possible than we might normally imagine. A belief in the promise of the human body, coupled with catalytic methods for evoking that promise, may unexpectedly bring vitality and healing to those resigned to unhappy fates. The potential is always lying dormant. We may be nicely surprised, startled, or sometimes, bowled over by its power.

One of the great blocks to becoming healthier is the lack of trust in the human body's talent for reorganizing itself. Just remembering this extraordinary talent and then activating it can change a life. When treatment methods bring about the seemingly impossible, they're not miraculous. They simply lie beyond the balustrades of the familiar. For example, in one type of acupuncture treatment, a needle inserted into the side of the right hand can instantly reduce or eliminate a certain type of pain in the left low back. This happens easily and routinely countless times a year throughout Asia, Europe, and the U.S. It's a normal and unsurprising result in acupuncture. If we're not familiar with CAM, it sounds nonsensical, impossible, or miraculous. It isn't miraculous at all. It's very ordinary and predictable—in its world.

What's been thought possible in our usual framework of medicine doesn't cover the whole landscape of possibility. Alternative and complementary medicine can mean the difference between health and illness for the millions of people yet to try it. In many cases, it could mean the difference between life and death. Those of us who are fortunate to do this work are gratified by seeing patients heal through the built-in brawn of their healing potential. But we can also be frustrated that this isn't practiced on a broader stage. If put to full use, much money can be saved and much suffering spared.

If our society isn't fully aware of CAM's potential, that doesn't qualify as an illusion in the way we've been using the word. But it does point to a big blind spot, a missed opportunity to nourish the health of the world.

The true diagnosis

Distortions, false assumptions, and biases not only contribute to poor health, but are, at times, the true diagnosis. A back pain may be the given diagnosis, with a code like 724.2, but the real diagnosis could be the illusion of being unloved. Another diagnosis might be blindness to the beauty within or the conviction that we are inadequate for our loved ones. We might have shoulder pain and asthma, but deep down, an existential loneliness within the marriage may lie at their roots. When we constrict the soul, our anguish or despondency may prevent the body from breathing freely.

Our distorted beliefs reflect what we most fear. And what we most fear is often what we most believe. The true diagnosis often lies in the roots of the tree of assumptions and illusions, not in the branches visible to the naked eye.

All this asks for our patience and courage in working through the layers of the symptoms. It can be time-consuming, confusing, laborious, even maddening. It can require the courage of Titans to face the pain inside and allow ourselves to be vulnerable. It's far easier to ask a professional for a medication, an herb, a homeopathic remedy, or an acupuncture treatment. Conversely, learning the most challenging of tasks—how to love ourselves and each other fully—leads to the opulence of the human soul, and therefore of the human body.

In one of the more poignant moments of the play *Our Town* by Thornton Wilder, the recently deceased Emily begs permission to leave the land of the dead for a brief return to her loved ones back on the earth. Ignoring the advice of her elders to stay put, she goes back to Grovers Corners, New Hampshire, for one more day.

Upon her return, she tells of being devastated by the blindness and ignorance afflicting those still on earth. They are too busy, too self-absorbed, she says, to see the beauty in front of them. During her time at home, she pleads with her mother to really look at her, to look into the soul of her daughter.

After returning, she asks the others among the dead if the living ever fully understand the depth of our humanness. In response, she gets a rant from neighbor Simon Stimson. He tells her of the cloud of ignorance that enshrouds people while they're alive, and how ignorance and self-centered passion lead them to hurt the feelings of others.

Wilder reminds us to respect the undercurrents of the soul lying behind appearances, just as Alan learned to do after surviving his aneurysm and close encounter with death.

When Wilder, Einstein, and the mystics write of illusions, they clearly refer to more than visual blocks. They suggest that breaking free of illusion makes us caring and compassionate. It's not just blindness to dark energy and dark matter or to mosquitoes in the dark, but to the illusion that love is absent. Being fully awake in this sense is not about an unfeeling perception. It's about being squarely positioned to see the love and benevolence that are always present in the world.

The predilection to be blind to the world's beauty is fed, in part, by fear. When the fear of loss, isolation, inadequacy, or rejection leads us to chase all that glitters, then it walls off the truly beautiful. The thrust of an indulgent culture pushes our interests toward the surface of living, like flotsam rising to the surface of the ocean.

The ripple and shimmer of the prosaic keep us myopic, unable to see the beautiful mysteries far below the surface. Behind any of these pursuits, we'll find the longing for what's meaningful and evocative, for what speaks to the soul. The expression of that longing is found in the everlasting appeal of art and literature where we find a contemporary mythology filled with parables about the luminosity of human character. But it's challenging to stay vigilant enough to see the veiled meaning and mystery under our very noses, every day and everywhere.

Among the chorales of religion, mysticism, and mythology, we hear repeatedly of a sacred and conscious Whole filled with meaning and purpose. The mystics and poets might say that though the faces of the gods are the handiwork of human dreams, what lies behind those faces is eternal, powerful, and meaningful.

Chapter Ten

Toward a Beautiful Medicine

Beauty is the splendor of truth

–Latin motto

Throughout the book, you may have found some of the ideas familiar and comfortable, or inspiring and informative, or perhaps radical, unnerving, confusing. Some of them are so foreign to our usual views of health and medicine that they can lead to philosophical heartburn. So before I describe what I mean by a beautiful medicine, a review of the main points may help.

Symptom as message

We started by looking at the usefulness of symptoms. They're not accidental, random sensations, but smart, logical messages from the wisdom of the mind and body. While the symptoms are certainly distressing, their strategy is benevolent. Historically, we've had it backward: we thought they were enemies, but they're friends. Since they're gruff coaches pushing us hard to play our best, we'll feel ruffled by their efforts. As annoying or devastating as symptoms can be, they're not problems. They're valuable instructions for change.

The Story of the Broken Window

To further explain the idea, the story of the broken window showed how many streams of influence converge, like rivers in a delta, to produce the symptom. These streams include our relationships, moods, financial pressures, lack of exercise, poor nutrition, and more. The story shows us that while the broken window is the most visible result, we must see the big picture to understand its source. The family does not have a window problem, and the baseball bat was not the cause of the broken window. But that's how we usually think of symptoms in our culture: each time a window breaks, we immediately think of ways to fix it or to remove bats.

The source of symptoms

Then we inquired into the ultimate origins of the symptom. We could say it came from the body, but then how did the phenomenon of human bodies come about in the first place? What's the genius behind the symptom's very existence? While the question may seem like conceptual gymnastics, it is crucial for understanding health better.

A pain is not just a pain. It's also the enigmatic, improbable intelligence of life bringing itself to life. It's part of the self-organizing ability of all life forms, found in the first creatures to crawl out of the sea. It's the sagacity expressed in every cell of billions of human bodies, in the bodies of all creatures from mosquito to whale. That sagacity is what you feel in pain and in every other possible sensation, whether through the five senses or in the mind.

In this light, then, the symptom is not merely personal, and not your individual property. Legally, yes, but existentially, no. It's much larger and older and consequential than that. This shift in viewpoints is heightened by remembering that you're never just sitting in a chair, but sitting on a planet in a universe.

A conscious universe

Next, we saw that mystics have been telling us for centuries that the world is spiritual in essence, and that some have said that consciousness is part of the universe itself. If we combine that with the idea that the symptom is a message, we could, ultimately, see symptoms as expressions of a conscious universe. Rumi wrote that our wounds are the place where the light enters us. That idea seems to find expression in the clinic where we can see a striking correspondence between the counsel of our spiritual teachers and behavior or emotions that have healing effects. We've long known that love and caring are good for the body, but now research supports this notion. Conversely, being stuck in chronic resentment, depression, resignation, or anxiety weakens the body.

The wellspring of healing

The next idea was that the subterranean wellspring of healing runs deep and strong. Its perseverance is remarkable, its vigor astonishing. We readily forget, or maybe never knew, that the source of healing is endogenous. Great resilience and stamina are available to those willing to draw upon that source of healing though exercise, a natural foods diet, and a peaceful, conscious heart. We can improve the odds even further with meaningful purpose, an inspired, joyful life, and a sturdy network of friends and family.

Control, substitute, catalyze

We then explored three categories of treatment strategies. The first is to *control*, which is necessary when the damage is serious enough that the body won't heal on its own. The second is to *substitute* for what the body might normally do on its own. The third is to *catalyze* the inherent potential for healing within the mind and body. These are three entirely different courses of action, each valuable for its intended purpose and not to be confused with the others. While the controlling and substitutive methods are essential for severe medical conditions, the catalytic methods have the advantage of helping us go from the absence of illness toward flourishing in body and soul. They draw upon the wellspring of human potential.

Health as transformation, medicine as catalyst

In Chapter Four, we looked at health as transformation. Health is more than the absence of disease, more than what's left after our symptoms are repaired. In this view, the perennial challenges of the human condition aren't appended to our physicality, but woven into its fibers. The grit of living, the endless unrest in our feet, and the encounters with those fates raising a fist against our happiness—all perpetually push us forward to find wholeness, precisely because of our feelings of repugnance toward them. In a reversal of our usual view of medicine's purpose, we can redefine this discomfort as a catalyst for the arc of psychological, social, and spiritual growth.

Symptoms teach us not only about corrections needed in the body, but about the most urgent of our psychological and spiritual concerns, including the shenanigans of the inner grinch or saboteur. Integrating the energies found in these and other shadowy elements of the self is essential for the evolution of character and wisdom. Symptoms then, whether physical or mental, are an integral part of the drama of the human experience. They emerge from the collective history of our genetic, familial, biological, and psychospiritual lives. They're simply part of the plan. This might have been what Nietzsche meant when he wrote that if it doesn't kill you, it will make you stronger.

The courage to heal

We then looked at fear as a purveyor of illness and at the medicinal properties of courage. Whether we're immobilized by a culture of indulgence or petrified by the dread of risk, our health suffers when we're frozen in fear. One common fear is that of feeling our emotions fully, and this includes the fear of grieving. But with the courage to let our tears come forth in a flood, we heal better. Conversely, repressing those tears builds pressure in the boiler room of the soul, which might then explode. The courage to assert, to risk, to grieve, to encounter, to break free of convention and inertia, to let off the steam—all help free the body's vitality and suppleness.

Meaning, purpose, and contribution in health

Chapter Six expanded on the idea that health is valuable not for itself, but for some other end. We value health for the freedom it gives us to pursue our passions. We looked at living with meaningful purpose as a source of energy. Meaning is itself energy, and at times, might so move you to attack a polar bear with your bare hands. Then, we heard from poets, playwrights, mystics, and psychiatrists asserting that the most gratifying of purposes is doing good for others. Contribution gives us energy and contentment, not necessarily as thrills at the five senses, but as an abiding sense of existential fullness. This sort of happiness, along with our healthy pleasures, helps us flourish.

Nourish and move

We then explored nutrition and exercise in their essence as nourishment and motion. Beyond their biological mechanics, we can see them as tools for becoming better synchronized with the architecture of human possibility.

Whole foods are information, teaching our cells to follow nature's playbook and so to grow toward optimum levels of performance. They help us evoke the powers of the earth and sea, fire and mountain, wind and tree. The same applies to motion: it persuades the inherent healing powers of mind and body to come out and dance.

The Whole

Here, we looked at the idea of the terrain as an essential idea in integrative medicine, as well as the broader idea of a Whole that includes all we can imagine and perhaps what lies beyond our imagination. In fact, the entire book has been pointing to the different faces of the Whole. Since some scientists believe that relationship is the fundamental building block of the universe, then the real DNA of life, the real subatomic particle, is not an undersized pellet but connectedness itself, relatedness itself. In other words, the physical world is made not of atoms, but of relationships—and this according to quantum physicists.

This then makes *relationship*, in its most essential and broadest philosophical sense, fundamental to health. We also saw that you can ache all over and feel wonderful, that how you feel overall is distinct from the state of your symptoms and a useful marker of health. For clinical purposes, as shown in the story of the broken window, we miss the point if we treat only the part and leave the terrain in disarray.

Awareness and healing

In Chapter Nine, we explored that connectedness further: mystics and some scientists have suggested that we live in the illusion of being separate from each other. We're deprived of vital energy when blind to our original intimacy with the world, to the recognition that not only are we blood relatives of all human beings, we're small but endogenous specks in the cosmic order. We normally see life distorted, as if looking through a dirty window, and that contributes to a sense of being split from the Whole. It doesn't mean that our world is unreal, but that we see it askew. This blurry world is more than just optical distortion.

As people from ancient Hindus to Einstein to Wilder have said, this distortion blinds us to the love and beauty in front of our noses. Dispelling the illusion of separateness leads to a kinder, healthier self. Many of our ailments are fed by the bitter taste of humiliation, the hollows of loneliness, the wounds of unspeakable loss, the unfulfilled yearning for a gentle touch on the arm. But weaving that straw into gold makes the body robust. By dissolving the illusions of alienation and isolation, we're made more whole.

This and other ideas throughout the book can be challenging to our usual perspectives because they don't fit into a neatly boxed worldview. They suggest that the world is more nuanced than it seems, more like a hologrammatic image through which we can run our hands. As most of the ideas are unorthodox, they paint a radically redefined picture of health and medicine that departs from the usual symbols of pill, scalpel, and hospital. But as we've seen throughout, becoming healthier is usually made easier if we look beyond, while including, the realm of flesh, organs, and bones. To truly understand health, we must include its psychological and philosophical dimensions. Otherwise, it's like trying to understand love by learning only the mechanics of sex.

So what's a beautiful medicine? Everything we've covered so far points to it. It's about the merger of science and art, truth and beauty, mind and soul with the biology of the fleshly body. It's the enfolding of our greatest hopes and deepest yearnings, the heart of the heart of our humanness, into a medicine that is deeper and broader than the customary. To start, let's first revisit the idea of the insistence—the evolutionary impulse.

The insistence

All theory aside, the will to happiness shows up as a conspicuous presence, an insistence, in the treatment room. The inflections in the voices of human drama seem to be informed by a primal compulsion that presses forward with the determination of a mother in search of her lost child. No matter the pursuit, whether it's for more money, power, love, or a piece of heaven, this insistence pushes us forward. Like the invisible marionette strings pulling birds, whales, and wildebeests in their migratory voyages, it's in a perpetual search for its final destination. While we have our individual versions of this drive, the impulse to acquire more and to become better is always there, even when it assumes destructive shapes. The desire for suicide is goal-seeking, too.

If we assume that the aggregate of human drama is informed by some sort of push to become more and to have more, can we explain it adequately by saying it's the biological drive of animal hungers in human clothing, that it's a more sophisticated version of survival of the fittest? That it so happened to get translated into art, literature, science, and spirituality? Many would say yes. Maybe meaning is just a convenience, mere sweat from neural gymnastics. Maybe the search for meaning is philosophical acrobatics that mollifies us with an illusion of significance.

On the other hand, we have mystics and philosophers throughout the centuries arguing for a meaningful universe. Given the mountain of books on the subject growing larger over the millennia, the refusal to consider this idea is an anti-intellectual snub. As we saw in earlier chapters, many of the brightest and most compassionate thinkers have suggested that this insistence, this intelligent drive, is the arc of an evolutionary impulse, signifying a universe that is not only physical but conscious as well.

Regardless of the arguments either way, a relentless human drive for wholeness shares the driver's seat with our distaste for suffering. No matter what we call it—the will to power, the survival instinct, the evolutionary impulse, the holy longing—we are thrust forward in pursuit, often pushed from behind by the hands of our symptoms.

To understand health in its essence, it helps to remember that we want it for reasons other than itself. To understand a hammer or screwdriver, we need to know their uses. Otherwise, they're wall hangings or doorstops. Similarly, purpose in health and medicine is essential to include in the big picture. If we get healthy, then what? Traditionally, that's where medicine stops and the so-called soft pursuits pick up—if you're not diseased, the line is drawn there. Then, leave it to the pastor, guru, imam, rabbi, to the poet or novelist, to the therapist or postmodern shaman to guide you in satisfying the urges that tingle in your toes—but don't leave it to medicine.

In contrast, I suggest that health and medicine are authentically meaningful only in light of our larger existential and spiritual questions. This takes us one step further toward the idea of a beautiful medicine.

A beautiful medicine

The task of understanding a beautiful medicine starts with seeing that everything occurs in context. We could even subtitle it contextual medicine. Context here includes the physical universe, and all relationships, art, morals, science—the works. It's easy to narrow our focus to what's in front of our noses, to forget that right now we're sitting in a chair in a universe tossed with trillions of stars. Where do you live? In the cosmos—a socially impractical though legitimate answer. This is not mysticism; it's science. Right now, you and I are moving at 67,000 miles an hour around the sun. That doesn't include the speed of the earth's rotation on its axis, or the speed at which our galaxy itself is moving through space, and other measures of different velocities. All told, we're moving through space in crossing rotations at a total of about

2,000,000 miles an hour without getting our latest haircut ruffled—a good reminder that all is not what it seems. It's essential to see broader contexts—an idea that we have covered throughout the book.

The search for a beautiful medicine gets a clue from poet John Keats who wrote:

> *Beauty is truth, truth beauty,—that is all*
> *Ye know on earth, and all ye need to know.*

It may not be the sum total of what we need to know, and love may not be all we need, as John Lennon wrote, but Keats does suggest an intriguing equivalence between truth and beauty. So here's a next step on the subject: this groundswell of insistence, this passion in our DNA, this heaving forward for more and better, could be seen as a force directing us toward the experience of beauty. Not the theory or idea of beauty, nor its objective meaning, but its direct subjective experience in our soul, skin, and bones.

We could define the final destination more philosophically, but what we want in our bones is to have it permeate us through and through. It's beauty not as an idea or as an abstraction, but as a palpable goodness and wholeness, of being moved to the core by joy and of being calmed by a sense of belonging. It's beauty we can sniff and taste, beauty as a destination where we find the fullest effusions of the human soul. From the perspective of what we really want, all theory aside, we could say that it's the experience of beauty—found in those moments when we're wholly in love with our children and spouses, and where everything adds up—where we feel we truly understand and belong. It all leads to this. These experiences are more than true; they're beautiful. They touch our core, the most impressionable fibers within, like the fingertips of seraphim stroking the soft, poignant spaces of the soul. At the very end, do we want knowledge and information, or do we want joy and gratification strong enough to lift us off the ground? I'm not at all arguing that this is a final answer to the larger existential and spiritual questions. It's more complex than this. But I am suggesting that from our subjective view, what we long to experience in the act of living is the perfume of love, beauty, and meaning—regardless of how it's defined philosophically, regardless of ideology.

Beauty heals

We can express this in other ways too. For example, it's been said that the entirety of human thought and discourse, everything that we have ever studied, can be put into the three groups of art, morals, and science—the beautiful, the good, and the true.

In that framework, what's missing in our current model of health is the art. Not art as in paintings and sculpture, but art in its essence showing up in the aesthetic, feeling experience of the authentic self. In medicine, the moral dimensions are clear. People practice medicine out of the concern for the wellbeing of others, and that sets the field on solid ground in that regard. The ethical violations in any health profession are deviations, not the norm. With regard to the science, it's clear that this is conventional medicine's strength. But a hole in medicine is left by the absence of art—the primacy of felt human experience, of the soul's interior, and in particular, the experience of beauty—again not art as in opera, painting, or ballet, but as that which is ineffable in the subjective, immeasurable part of our humanness.

In the end, it's that felt sense, not just an idea, that calls to us. It's that part of us where the heart is disarmed by the radiance and innocence of our squeaky little children, upon realizing how loyal our friends and family have been, upon having our breath taken away when walking into a cathedral with medieval stained glass, or into an incense-filled stone temple in India, or into a Zen garden in Kyoto. It's this felt experience, regardless of any rational definitions of where we're ultimately going, regardless of the loftiness of our philosophical language, that draws us forward.

A beautiful medicine honors all the faces of human endeavor, including the brilliance and necessity of hard scientific data as bedrock. But it emphasizes that in the end, each patient and each healthcare provider wants to discover the soul of human experience. This is not antiscientific, but transcientific. A trans-Atlantic flight is not anti-Atlantic.

Going beyond the popular notion that an integrative medicine is a combination of conventional and holistic methods, a beautiful medicine is integrative in all ways and includes the richness of the poetic self—an appreciation of love, awe, and wonder— as a core element of health even when we are surrounded by scalpels, whirring machines, and medication dripping through a tube into an arm. It breathes and pulses as a living medicine informed by the endless longing that pulls us toward wholeness.

Different kinds of truth

If, as the Latin motto goes, beauty is the splendor of truth, or if beauty is truth and truth beauty according to Keats, we have a curious equation. At the least, we can listen to the voices of the great artists and scientists who suggest that science is not the only avenue to truth. The arts, in their eyes, are also a search for truth, though for truth with a different face.

The aesthetic impulse is more than the lust for gratification or for charming the senses. As Eros, it brings us much more than sex. What musicians, artists, actors, and writers seek through it is mercurial, but when it arrives under dazzling lights, it moves us, kissing us at the core. This gives us better coordinates for discovering where and how we fit on the map. The mission of a beautiful medicine is to call upon this other type of truth while still paying due respect to the quantitative strengths of the scientific method.

The experience of *I am* is a type of truth. Feeling fully oneself—awake, alive, and aware—is a kind of truth that can't be quantified. When brought to tears by the kindness of our children or through ecstasy with a lover, we would be unhinged to think of testing the experiences for their truth or falsehood. This type of truth comes in those occasional moments when the gates of a concealed world open wide as we gaze at a rose and violet dusk at Taos, smell the elegance of jasmine, or see in another's eyes the love we've always desired. At those times when we dive under the surface into the authentic self, we know in our bellies that we do belong here. But more often than not, we drift in the whirlpool of conflicting desires, pressured glances, and vague anxieties.

Picasso asked, "Are we to paint what's on the face, what's inside the face, or what's behind it?" Clearly, art was truth seeking to him, leading him to look for the silent, invisible worlds lying behind a flower or a face. His genius and that of the master artists lay, in part, in the ability to see the through the veils, to trust that flowers and faces were doorways to a hidden world both opulent and occasionally terrifying. He might have agreed with Iris Murdoch, who wrote:

> *Love is the extremely difficult realization that something other than oneself is real. Love, and so art and morals, is the discovery of reality.*

In the same vein, Rollo May wrote:

> *What if imagination and art are not frosting at all, but the fountainhead of human experience? What if our logic and science derive from art forms and are fundamentally dependent on them rather than art being merely a decoration for our work when science and logic have produced it?*

Years earlier, Albert Einstein wrote:

> *How can cosmic religious feeling be communicated from one person to*

another if it can give rise to no definite notion of a God and no theology?
In my view, it is the most important function of art and science to awaken
this feeling and keep it alive in those who are receptive to it.

In a reversal of how a scientific culture views imagination and art, Einstein, the penultimate scientist, lays out his priorities: both science and art are here for the purpose of awakening religious feeling. Rollo May suggests that logic and science are derived from art—which he says is not decoration but the very source of human experience. He has suggested a radical view for our time, and in doing so, he assigns to science a role that is secondary to art and morals, much in accord with Einstein's thoughts.

On this relationship between beauty and truth, Hans-Georg Gadamer, in one sentence, captured the essence of what I've been attempting to say when he wrote, "...the experience of the beautiful, and particularly the beautiful in art, is the invocation of a potentially whole and holy order of things, wherever it may be found."

To think of beauty as one face of truth may seem unusual, as the industrialized world has been dominated by stiffer realities. But throughout the millennia, the relentless pursuit of truth and beauty through art has shown no signs of abating, and that tenacity is itself noteworthy.

Whether in the form of paintings, songs, or books infused by the creators' naked humanness, or on the runways of fashion and in the flashbulb fascination with celebrity, we continue in that pursuit. From the cave paintings at Lascaux 40,000 years ago to the genius of James Joyce, Georgia O'Keefe, and Luciano Pavarotti, we continue the undying search for a meaningful ethos, for the heaven-worlds that can be seen only by the lucid eye. That this search exists at all is itself a form of evidence.

One of the most poignant moments of my life came when truth and beauty intersected on Christmas Day of 1982. I was at my parents' house in northern Virginia. After breakfast and the morning gift exchange, my mother turned to preparing dinner, and since I had little else to do, I went outside on the sunny and unseasonably warm day to tinker with the engine of my red Volkswagen Beetle.

I had returned to live in the Washington area after my time in Sri Lanka because my father was suffering from congestive heart failure. Since he'd already suffered two heart attacks, I wanted to live nearby in case I was needed. After I'd been working on the engine for a while, he came out of the house to see how I was doing—the father with whom I'd argued and fought endlessly during my teen years, who had never once said "I love you," whose hands had not once embraced his boys and had too often smacked their butts when they were young.

He was a funny, loyal father with sandpaper edges, no high school diploma, and the emotional dents from growing up poor in Quebec. Although a dedicated father, his good intentions for order and control among his three sons had been no match for rowdy teen spirit. This often triggered his volcanic temper. His voice, often getting brutish and edgy, was always five decibels too loud even in normal conversation.

Fortunately, he and I had gotten along much better in recent years, starting the day he left me on my first day of college. As he prepared to drive back home, I relished the thought of finally being free of parental rule. But when we shook hands and said goodbye, his eyes got moist. I was dumbfounded. This meant that somewhere in his boot-camp heart were affections for me I hadn't known about, and from that moment on, the history of our relationship, as I knew it, was rewritten. It was the first step toward our healing. Over the years, he softened further, and for my part, I became more tolerant of his hardened ways. But we still had never said "I love you" to each other. That would have been awkward and unmanly. It was easier to argue politics.

For a few minutes, we talked about the engine. Maybe it was about the carburetor or the valves, I don't remember. But it was pleasant, casual talk.

Suddenly, as I looked past his bifocals into his sharp blue eyes, something in them shifted, and something between us woke up. I could see, I just knew, that he loved me. The look was unmistakable. And I could see that he knew I loved him too. He looked forgiven. For a few seconds, the rest of the world vanished, and we were fused in this beautiful brilliant intimacy, seeing and knowing each other as though for the first time. As we stood there flooded with grace, looking into each other's eyes, the pain and doubts of a lifetime with him were lifted off my shoulders. I trusted that he too felt complete as he approached the end of his life, knowing that I loved him and forgave him. The only words we spoke aloud were about carburetors and valves. Six days later on New Year's Eve, in the middle of the night, my father's heart stopped beating for the last time.

No scientific tests will validate the truth of that christening between us. Those few fleeting seconds redefined the meaning of my relationship with him in a truth that is known only to art, morals, and soul, a truth that can grow in the well-composted soil of the human narrative—only in the language of the beautiful and the good. How could we quantify that? It's a truth, a beautiful truth, that has rung its redemptive tones throughout my life since then.

When the doors of perception are thrown wide open, we carry with us, to the end, the adornments of beauty and truth merged into a seamless whole. These are truths of a different variety, and essential to the notion of a beautiful medicine.

Our culture is prejudiced against seeking truth with the aesthetic eye. This sort of prejudice toward what we can't measure and control has distorted our views of medicine and health. Today, no diagnostic code exists for the soreness caused by the lack of beauty or inspiration. No procedure code exists for the healing power of compassion or forgiveness. For all its towering strengths and miraculous work, a mechanistic view of medicine that sees the human body as on object to be engineered gives us a fragment of the whole picture. And incomplete truths can be misleading, sometimes dangerous. If we treat a man's painful shoulder and ignore his broken heart, whether as a massage therapist, acupuncturist, or surgeon, we see only the part, not the whole.

Practically speaking, health professionals can't be all things to all people. But they can be renaissance clinicians adapted to twenty-first century sensibilities, and practice a beautiful medicine by being aligned with the patient's grandest hopes and quietest longings—by catching the drift of the whole Kafkaesque narrative behind the spot that hurts. They can think of medication, herbs, surgery, vitamins, and secular incantations as tools that ultimately serve the purpose of nurturing those hopes and longings. They can practice a medicine that welcomes the human soul into the domicile of hard science—an approach that can be practiced anywhere by any type of health professional, regardless of technique.

The practice of medicine can be a living, breathing human encounter that enlivens the soul of the patient, whether through an ancient herb, a pharmaceutical cocktail, the laying-on of hands, a razor-sharp scalpel, or a prayer. Since health is for something else, medicine's end purpose must also be something other than itself. It doesn't exist for its own sake. It's just another tool for helping us along on the search for that elusive sense of actualization, for wholeness in the soul, for learning how to love fully—for doing what springtime does to cherry trees.

A beautiful medicine, as defined here, includes forever dispelling the notion that health is just physical and medicine only remedial. It speaks of the radiance behind human experience showing itself through the symptoms, of seeing Rumi's idea that a blinding, unearthly light is trying to enter us through the bandaged place.

Rumi wrote that the truth emerges thorough our wounds. Rilke wrote of the god wanting to know himself in you. Buber wrote that when a person listens to the *great will, he listens to what grows*—to a message being formed out of the void. The vibrancy of what lies beyond our conscious selves, the *insistence*, is always seeking expression, however painful it may be on occasion.

Buber also insisted that the *great will* needs us and wants to be actualized by us, *with human spirit and human deed, with human life and human death.* How refreshing to think that we're needed by the fates, when in contrast, we usually ask them for help. We call on them in times of our need, asking for intervention against the wicked or unjust blows of destiny. We may find ourselves reoriented in the world by the peculiar thought that destiny needs us too.

Does this mean that every health professional must have a long conversation about meaning, purpose, and soul with each patient? Not at all. But practitioners of any type of medicine can remember that while the form of their work might be treatment of the body, *what they are essentially and always treating is the patient's humanness.* Whether the diagnosis is a sore knee or leukemia, the tools a handful of dandelion greens or a $2 million surgical robot, they can be mindful that the patient is playing out a personal story full of slings and arrows with fortunes hallowed or outrageous. The practitioners can remember that within each transient, recyclable human body lie the blessings of the wind and fire, the earth and sea, the sun and moon—all blended in an alchemical cauldron of possibility. Whether or not they help a person with more than the broken part will depend on their time, clinical training, and inclinations. But they can always remember that they're treating what's invisible and meaningful—the rich core of the patient's humanness— even while bandaging a cut, excising a tumor, or massaging a neck.

This is not to imply that all integrative medicine, or CAM, embodies this ideal and that conventional medicine does not. In fact, most holistic or integrative approaches are still focused on treating the physical self without considering the deeper humanism, the human spirit in the biological self. This vision of the humanism within the body is often absent in schools of holistic medicine as well as in medical schools. On the other hand, many nurses, like Barbara Dossey and Jean Watson, and many physicians, like Larry Dossey, Christiane Northrup, Deepak Chopra, and Bernie Siegel, advocate a deeper understanding of the holism of medicine. My friends who are physicians and nurses are dedicated, compassionate people with big hearts and sensitive souls, well aware of holism. Whether we administer valerian root or valium, St. John's wort or anti-depressants, what matters is to honor the humanity of the patient. It does not depend on the type of medicine practiced.

Full circle

It came roundabout for me. In the end, much of what I was looking for in Sri Lanka was given me by my work as a health professional. In the idealism and romanticism of the late sixties and early seventies, the glamour of faraway exotic lands seemed to hold a promise unavailable at home. And though I looked for my dream in the clouds, in the end, I found it at my feet.

My laboratory was not to be the monastery, but a normal life where I had to learn how to better love family and friends, to grapple with the challenges of parenting, to better listen to my patients year after year after year. I saw that the prize was in the immediacy of the daily grind, and that my spiritual practices were ultimately occupational training for my personal life. Over time, my get-spiritual-quick approach made way for a slower ripening, a curve of learning that included changing diapers and washing dishes and mowing the lawn. I see more clearly that life is improv, where I learn from the blunders that must come when ad-libbing on the stage of our eminently human everyday dramas. I find it supremely ironic that this full encounter and presence in the here-and-now is what meditation teaches us in the first place.

I had gotten trapped in looking forward to being in the present moment.

Listening to my patients over the years has been an extraordinary, humbling experience. By virtue of my role as a health professional, I've been endowed with the sacred trust of listening to my patients' stories of sorrow, rage, or betrayal, and their tales of hushed, secret pains. My position has slowly shaped and molded me over nearly three decades, toward what I'd hoped to become by meditating for a couple of years on a jewel of a tropical island. Being a professional caregiver elicits the altruistic self merely through the structure of the work, through the expectations of how we are to behave. Over the years, it can chisel and sculpt character, one success and one embarrassment at a time. It's only in retrospect that the work's influence in shaping character becomes evident.

When we put ourselves in a supportive role, we bypass our personal concerns—if only temporarily. After all, the client or patient is not paying to hear about the caregiver's troubles. It's an opportunity for the professional to be reminded that it's not all about him. In one Non Sequitur cartoon, a small, frightened man in shackles stands before a chopping block. Next to the block stands a hulking man in a black hood, holding a giant axe, ready to behead the prisoner. He looks sardonically at the trembling prisoner and says, "Oh right…it's all about you, isn't it?" In simple terms, one of the most gratifying of human tasks is to have learned that it's not all about you.

Year after year, I've sat in the listening seat whether I was energetic or lethargic, focused or distracted, attentive or self-absorbed, calm or restless. With the slightest decency, the human response in these circumstances is to shift the focus to the person sitting in the other chair. Since the script calls for us to be helpful, we act accordingly. It's not a matter of character, but of training. The more we train, the more the habits become ingrained.

Ancient spiritual texts don't mention embarrassment, powerlessness, and humiliation in the social encounter as antidotes for egocentrism. But in the laboratory of the daily social or professional exchange, they work well.

In the earliest years of civilization, there was little psychology apart from spirituality, so the approach to growth and development back then was mostly esoteric, contemplative, or ritualistic. We were to grow through devotion, prayer, and meditation. But in the end, and as some of the teachings insist, I've found that the esoterics of our spiritual lessons are right in front of our eyes. The lofty invocations, the exotic scents and statues, and the soaring hymns all point to what's already in front of us.

I've learned the most from the constant imprecisions in the human encounter. Again, this is what many spiritual teachings tell us in the first place, captured famously in William Blake's lines that we can find the world in a grain of sand and heaven in a wildflower. I've learned much from the professor, author, and spiritual teacher, but I've also learned from the kindness in a grandma's voice and the pure sweetness of a toddler's smile.

Parenthood has also shaped me for the better. For one thing, the ambiguities in the improbable task of balancing love with discipline is a most humbling experience. I found parenting to involve constant tacking as we would in a sailboat, though I suspect that in sailing, the tack is usually rewarded with a little more certainty about having done the right thing.

In parenting, that knowledge won't come until the child is grown, and even then, you're never quite sure. But one privilege of parenthood is that it's temporary custody of a human being who is one small measure of the fecundity of life itself. I think of the job of parenting as the donation of alms to the grand scheme of the evolutionary impulse, one charming, adoring, twinkling set of eyes at a time. We raise not just a child, but one part of the brilliant Whole. The love I have for my children has repositioned me in my world and has been priceless for my personal evolution. As with being a caregiver, we tend to rise to the occasion, putting other before self...what we wouldn't do to protect our children from harm. If yielding to the allure of our indulgences means our child won't have new shoes for school, we'll reconsider. In the end, parenting is a superb testing ground for what all our spiritual teachings call for: patience, forgiveness, empathy, compassion.

Then there's the sensation of being suspended in midair that comes from knowing we're powerless. Our children are their own people, and, once grown, we can't stop them from running into the street without looking. We still try, of course, which may be the root of most conflicts between parent and child. Though all we want is the best for them, that desire itself leads to tension, however necessary and inevitable, if we are to be a parent at all.

In my case, I suspect that my adult children now just think, *Okay, there goes Dad spouting off again, addicted to giving advice, so we'll nod politely, ignore it, and let him be his fogey old self.* They're mature enough now to see through a parent's overinflated worries and well-intentioned meddling, unlike the gullible years when they swallowed whole our stories about Santa. This helps me get my coordinates on the map, seeing that I've moved into a phase of my life that's more about passing on the torch, about soon making way for the brain and muscle of the coming generations. Between monkhood and parenthood, the latter was my destiny, and I'm deeply grateful.

And in the end

There's a delicate line between the psychological and the spiritual, and it can show up through the love we have for each other, in the breathing, pulsing I-You encounter described by Martin Buber. When we are deeply, profoundly in love with our children, lovers, or spouses, the sheer energy of that love can take us deep enough that we drop into the realms of the sacred. At that point, it may no longer be just personal, human love, but a brushing up against the flickering edges of mystery itself. We can, at times, come to those edges through our very human love for another, where the other soul becomes a doorway into the chambers where *agape* and *eros* are blended into one. In this place, in the fusion of mind and soul, we can begin to drop our past, our masks, and our boundaries. In the end, a beautiful medicine supports us in that quest.

T.S. Eliot wrote that we will not cease from exploration—an idea that is reminiscent of the evolutionary impulse, of the *blessed unrest*, and of Goethe's *holy longing*. He may have had in mind the human desire endlessly insistent on driving us in search of actualization. Eliot also wrote that we will end up where we started, knowing the place for the first time—a place of Zen simplicity and nothingness—but with a different set of eyes to see who we truly are for the first time. I believe that line captures the full circle of my life, from the longings of my earlier years to the sense of fulfillment I have today. The thin line between the mind and soul, between the ordinary and the fantastic, can be found right here between you and me.

In "Little Gidding," Eliot writes:

> *We shall not cease from exploration*
> *And the end of all our exploring*
> *Will be to arrive where we started*
> *And know the place for the first time.*
> *Through the unknown, unremembered gate*
> *When the last of earth left to discover*
> *Is that which was the beginning;*
> *At the source of the longest river*
> *The voice of the hidden waterfall*
> *And the children in the apple-tree*
> *Not known, because not looked for*
> *But heard, half-heard, in the stillness*
> *Between two waves of the sea.*

Quick now, here, now, always—

A condition of complete simplicity

(Costing not less than everything)

And all shall be well and

All manner of thing shall be well

When the tongues of flames are in-folded

Into the crowned knot of fire

And the fire and the rose are one.

A beautiful medicine is the integration of all that we know of love, healing, and health in a blended singularity. It points to those moments, which most of us have known, that take us beyond ourselves into an exquisite place that is at once human and divine. To love someone in that timeless space between heaven and earth, to look into the eyes of a child and see the shimmering of beauty, to know that she is an eternal yes, or that she is the past, present, and future unfolding all at once in a diaphanous loving luminosity, is to glimpse our own full humanness. In those moments, we sense that those sweet eyes— whether of our child, lover, spouse, or parent—are portals to the heart of hearts. We look not into their eyes, but past them into a pulsing, thrumming yes enveloping us in boundless warmth. Do all roads of human effort lead toward this one thin spot where two worlds meet, this one heart, a threshold of the radiant? At this place, we are thrust headfirst through a narrow opening for a new birth, a beginning so beautiful that our pretenses dissolve in its pure endless waters, leaving us wholly exposed.

Ultimately, can medicine be seen anew as a discipline helping us inch closer, as far as we can, toward this greater wholeness? Is medicine just for fixing problems in the body, or for serving as one of many endeavors that help us become fully awake? Is this precious ground of healing another clinical commodity for improved statistical outcomes, or is it what statistical analyses and research data should bow to, hands to the forehead, all the way to the ground?

This pulsing between two hearts in a love equaling wisdom is an omega point, the place we reach at the end of our labors and our weeping, of our small, short deaths of anguish and downward glances—all of which were driven in the first place by the fiery insistence that reaches from the place between our legs up to the brain of the heart and then to the heart of the brain and then to the sky. The inexhaustible yearning, the urge to fuse with another human soul, the longing to be touched by the effusions of another heart, or the desperation to cross the chasm of loneliness, to avoid the crush of humiliation, to hunt for imperturbable peace—was all this just love pushing us from behind, speaking in soft but unyielding tones? If we can fully know ourselves for the first time, then the bursting of the seams of the self happens in a crescendo, at the omega point of splendor, meaning, and the heart's full satiety. It was all already there, waiting, waiting, for us to finally arrive and understand.

References

Introduction

Bellow, Saul. *Humboldt's Gift*. New York: Penguin Books, 1996.
Swimme, Brian. *The Universe is a Green Dragon*. Rochester: Bear & Company, 2001.
Cummings, E.E. *A Selection of Poems*. New York: Harcourt Brace Jovanovich, 1965.

Chapter One

The Spirit of Medicine: The Old, the New, and the Beautiful

Judy Garland: from "My Love is Lost," in a privately published book of poems. Judy
Garland Database, http://www.jgdb.com/jgbk7.htm.
Of all the healers....Hormoz Ebrahimnejad, "Religion and Medicine in Iran: from
Relationship to Dissociation." *Hist. Sci.*, xl (2002).
When the minds of the people are closed....*The Yellow Emperor's Classic of Internal
Medicine*, trans. Ilza Veith. Berkely: University of California Press, 1972.
There is no house....David Whyte, from *The House of Belonging*. Langley: Many
Rivers Press, 2010.

Chapter Two

The Symptom as Message

Walt Whitman, from "Leaves of Grass" in *Walt Whitman, The Complete Poems*.
London, Penguin Books, 2004.
Chronic disease....the Centers for Disease Control (CDC) estimated in 2009 that
greater than 75% of chronic diseases are preventable. "Chronic Diseases: The
Power to Prevent, The Call to Control: At A Glance 2009" http://www.cdc.gov/
chronicdisease/resources/publications/AAG/chronic.htm.
The world is only spiritual....p. 246, from *Talks with Ramana Maharshi*. Carlsbad,
CA: Inner Directions, 2001.
Coex....Stanislav Grof, M.D with Hal Zina Bennett, *The Holotropic Mind*. New York:
HarperCollins, 1993.
The individual is an aperture....Alan Watts, *The Art of Contemplation*. New York:
Pantheon Books, 1972.
Brian Swimme, *Op.cit.*
Love is the affinity....Pierre Teilhard de Chardin, *Activation of Energy*. London:
William Collins Sons & Co., 1970.
Don't look at the bandaged place....from *The Essential Rumi*, translations by Coleman
Barks with John Moyne. San Francisco: HarperCollins, 1995.

Chapter Three
The Wellspring of Healing

Truly being here is glorious. Rainer Maria Rilke, *The Selected Poetry of Rainer Maria Rilke*, ed. and trans. by Stephen Mitchell. New York: Vintage Books, 1984.

Ann: During an interview in 2010, Ann's oncologist told me that the diagnosis of stage IV small cell lung cancer in the right lung was made in June 2008 when Ann was 86 years old. The mass of about 1.5 cm was confirmed initially by X-ray and later with a CAT scan. The scan also showed widespread metastases to the lymph nodes. A PET scan later that month showed evidence that the cancer had spread to the bones, most notably to her ribs and upper back. A mass of 2.5 cm was also detected in her right hip. While no biopsy of the suspected bone metastases was performed, the appearance was clearly consistent with bone cancer.

After the June diagnosis, Ann received two cycles of carboplatin and etoposide in July, but with significant side effects. The chemotherapy was therefore stopped. Then in August, she was administered rounds of cisplatin and irinotecan, again with significant side effects, so that regimen was also stopped. Additionally, she was administered zometa, a bone builder.

In addition to the chemotherapy, Ann also received acupuncture, massage, acupressure, and hypnotherapy. She prayed, meditated, took supplements as recommended by a naturopath, and ate healthily.

By October 8, 2008, the scans showed no sign of bone cancer. The large mass in her right hip was gone, and a CAT scan of her lungs showed that the tumor had shrunk to 0.8 cm. All the lymph nodes were clear. For people of any age, the chances of survival with a stage IV lung cancer are close to nothing, and for Ann, in her eighties, they were a step away from impossible. The oncologist said, "I've never seen anyone like her."

Staggering news about the body's intrinsic healing potential: some cancers, in the early stages, vanish of their own accord, i.e. without treatment: "Rethinking Screening for Breast Cancer and Prostate Cancer," *Journal of the American Medical Association*. 2009;302(15):1685-1692. Ann's stage IV cancer, however, was highly advanced, and a reversal was improbable.

Centenarians: http://en.wikipedia.org/wiki/Centenarians.

Dan Buettner, *The Blue Zones*. Washington DC: National Geographic Society, 2008.

Chapter Four
Health as Transformation, Medicine as Catalyst

Langston Hughes. *The Collected Poems of Langston Hughes*, Arnold Rampersad, editor, David Roessel, Associate Editor. New York: Vintage, 2004.
States and stages....Ken Wilber, *Integral Spirituality*. Boston: Shambala, 2006.
Joseph Campbell, *The Hero with a Thousand Faces*. Princeton: Princeton University Press, 1973.

Chapter Five
The Courage to Heal

Prevalence of diabetes in 2050: Boyle, James P, et al. "Projection of the Year 2050 Burden of Diabetes In the US Adult Population: Dynamic Modeling of Incidence, Mortality, and Prediabetes Prevalence," *Population Health Metrics* 2010, 8:29 doi:10.1186/1478-7954-8-29.
The impact of poverty on health: Nortin M. Hadler, M.D., *The Last Well Person—How to Stay Well Despite the Healthcare System*. Montreal-Kingston: McGill-Queen's University Press, 2004.
Broken-heart syndrome: Movahed MR, Donohue D., Review: transient left ventricular apical ballooning, broken heart syndrome, ampula cardiomyopathy, atypical apical ballooning, or Tako-Tsubocardiomyopathy. *Cardiovasc Revasc Med.* 2007 Oct-Dec;8(4):289-92.
"Broken heart" syndrome: real, potentially deadly but recovery quick: http://www.hopkinsmedicine.org/press_releases/2005/02_10_05.html.
Normal Mailer, *The Spooky Art: Some Thoughts on Writing*. New York: Random House, 2003.
Mary F. Dallman, et al., *Chronic Stress and Obesity: A New View of "Comfort Food."* 11696—11701, PNAS. September 30, 2003, vol. 100, no. 20.
Deborah Tannen, Ph.D., *That's Not What I Meant*. New York: Ballantine Books, 1986.
Give sorrow words....William Shakespeare, *Macbeth*.
Nine times as much TV watching and other leisurely activities than on exercise.... Linda Dong, Gladys Block, Shelly Mandel, *Activities Contributing to Total Energy Expenditure in the United States: Results from the NHAPS Study*. International Journal of Behavioral Nutrition and Physical Activity, 2004, 1:4 doi:10.1186/1479-5868-1-4.

Chapter Six

Meaning, Purpose, and Health

"Inuit See Signs in Arctic Thaw; String of Warm Winters Alarms 'Sentries for the Rest of the World.'" Doug Struck, *The Washington Post*; Mar 22, 2006; A.01

Martin Buber, *I and Thou*. New York: Charles Scribner and Sons, 2003.

Viktor E. Frankl, *Man's Search for Meaning*. Boston, Beacon Press, 1992.

George Bernard Shaw, *Man and Superman—A Comedy and a Philosophy*. Charleston: CreateSpace, 2010.

Mihaly Csikszentmihalyi, *Flow—The Psychology of Optimal Experience*. New York: HarperCollins, 1990.

George Leonard and Michael Murphy, *The Life We Are Given*. New York: Jeremy P. Tarcher/Putnam, 1995.

Martin Buber, *Op.cit.*

Stanislav Grof, M.D., *The Cosmic Game*. Albany: State University of New York Press, 1995.

Helen Schuchman, *A Course in Miracles: Combined Volume*. Mill Valley: Foundation for Inner Peace, 2007.

The god wants to know himself in you.....*The Collected Poetry of Rainer Maria Rilke*, ed. & trans. by Stephen Mitchell. New York: Vintage, 1984.

Dopamine, rats....Wise RA. "Brain Reward Circuitry: Insights from Unsensed Incentives." *Neuron*. 2002; 36:229-340.

Olds J. "Self-Stimulation of the Brain." *Science. 1958; 127:315-324.*

Purpose as an act of declaration....my exposure to this idea came indirectly from Martin Heidegger through the work of philosopher Fernando Flores, who in turn influenced the work of Landmark Educational Corporation.

Free is the man....Martin Buber, *Op.cit.*

James Joyce, *A Portrait of the Artist as a Young Man*. London: Penguin Modern Classics, 1972.

CaringBridge: www.caringbridge.org.

Chapter Seven

Nourish: The Breath of Flowers

Institute for Functional Medicine: www.functionalmedicine.org

Nutrigenomics....Gerald Rimbach, Jurgen Fuchs (ed), *Nutrigenomics: Oxidative Stress and Disease*. CRC Press, 2005. From the book description: "Nutritional genomics, also referred to as nutrigenomics, is considered one of the next frontiers in the post-genomic era. Its fundamental premise is that while alterations in gene expression or epigenetic phenomena can subvert a healthy phenotype into manifesting chronic disease, through the introduction of certain nutrients, this process can be reversed or modified. Employing state-of-the-art genomic and proteomic investigations that monitor the expression of thousands of genes in response to diet, nutrigenomics investigates the occurrence of relationship between dietary nutrients and gene expression." Epigenetics...."John Cloud, Why Your DNA Isn't Destiny." *Time Magazine*, January 2010. http://www.time.com/time/magazine/article/0,9171,1952313,00.html. Epigenetics....Eva Jablonka, *Evolution in Four Dimensions: Genetic, Epigenetic, Behavioral, and Symbolic Variation in the History of Life*. Boston: The MIT Press, 2006.

Caloric restriction.... "Scientists Ferret out a Key Pathway for Aging," ScienceDaily.com, Nov.18,2010. http://www.sciencedaily.com/releases/2010/11/101118124201.htm.

For nearly sixty years, scientists have consistently found that caloric restriction increases longevity in animals. Some more recent studies have begun to question that link, but a large body of evidence supports the idea.

DNA and destiny.....John Cloud, Why Your DNA Isn't Your Destiny." *Time Magazine*, Jan. 06, 2010. http://www.time.com/time/magazine/article/0,9171,1952313,00.html.

Water intake...The Institute of Medicine recommends 91 ounces of water a day for women, and 125 ounces for men. However, this includes water in all beverages and in food such as fruit and vegetables. Institute of Medicine, *Dietary Reference Intakes for Water, Potassium, Sodium, Chloride, and Sulfate*. Washington, D.C.: National Academies Press, 2005.

For an entirely different view on the need for water, see F. Batmanghelidj, *Your Body's Many Cries for Water*. Global Health Solutions, Inc.,2008. The author states that chronic dehydration is prevalent and a contributor to many ailments.

Christopher Crowley & Henry S. Lodge, M.D., *Younger Next Year—A Guide to Living Like 50 Until You're 80 and Beyond*. New York: Workman Publishing, 2004. The authors recommend exercising six days a week for the rest of your life, including serious aerobic exercise four times a week, and serious strength training two times a week.

Fitness and academics in Naperville School District, California Board of Education.... John J. Ratey, M.D., with Eric Hagerman. *Spark—the Revolutionary New Science of Exercise and the Brain*. New York: Little, Brown and Company, 2008.

Recommended exercise levels: Institute of Medicine, *Dietary Reference Intakes for Energy, Carbohydrate, Fiber, Fat, Fatty Acids, Cholesterol, Protein, and Amino Acids*. Washington, D.C.: National Academies Press, 2002.

Exercise reduced the incidence of all-cause mortality in men...the more vigorous the exercise, the greater the reduction in risk of death. I-Min Lee et al., *Exercise Intensity and Longevity in Men. Journal of the American Medical Association*. 1995;273:1179-1184.

Chapter Eight
The Whole

Vlatko Vedral, *Decoding Reality: The Universe as Quantum Information.* New York: Oxford University Press, USA, 2010.

Rosengren A, et al, "Association of psychosocial risk factors with risk of acute myocardial infarction in 11119 cases and 13648 controls from 52 countries (the INTERHEART study): case-control study." *Lancet.* 2004 Sep 11-17;364(9438):953-62.

Yusuf S, et al, on behalf of the INTERHEART Study Investigators. "Effect of potentially modifiable risk factors associated with myocardial infarction in 52 countries (the INTERHEART study): case-control study." *Lancet.* 2004;364:937-952.

David S. Sheps, MD, et al. "The INTERHEART Study: Intersection Between Behavioral and General Medicine." *Psychosomatic Medicine* 66:797-798 (2004).

Chapter Nine
Aware, Awake, Alive

Dark matter, dark energy....Richard Panek, "Probing the Biggest Mystery in the Universe." *Smithsonian:* April 2010 Volume 41, Number 1.

Humberto R. Maturana and Franciso J. Varela, *The Tree of Knowledge—the Biological Roots of Human Understanding.* Boston: Shambala Press, 1988.

Chapter Ten
Toward a Beautiful Medicine

Rollo May, *The Courage to Create.* New York: Bantam Books, 1980.

Hans-Georg Gadamer, *The Relevance of the Beautiful and Other Essays.* Cambridge: Cambridge University Press, 1986.

281

A Beautiful Medicine

Resources

Academic Consortium for Complementary and Alternative Healthcare,
    http://www.accahc.org/
American Academy of Osteopathy, http://www.academyofosteopathy.org/
American Association of Naturopathic Physicians, http://www.naturopathic.org/
American Chiropractic Association, http://www.acatoday.org/
American Herbalists Guild, http://www.americanherbalistsguild.com/
American Nutrition Association, http://americannutritionassociation.org/
American Massage Therapy Association, http://www.amtamassage.org/index html
The Bravewell Collaborative: Transforming Healthcare and Improving the Health of
    the Public Through Integrative Medicine, http://www.bravewell.org/
Consortium of Academic Health Centers for Integrative Medicine,
    http://www.imconsortium.org/
The Integrator Blog, http://theintegratorblog.com/
National Center for Complementary and Alternative Medicine (NCCAM),
    http://nccam.nih.gov/
National Center for Homeopathy, http://www.homeopathic.org/
National Commission for the Certification of Acupuncture and Oriental Medicine,
    http://www.nccaom.org/
Samueli Institute—Exploring the Science of Healing, http://www.siib.org/

For a free download of
The Beautiful Medicine Discovery Guide,
visit
www.abeautifulmedicine.com or
www.davidgmercier.com

The Discovery Guide focuses on practical steps you can take to implement the principles of *A Beautiful Medicine*. In contrast to the book itself, which emphasizes key concepts, the *Discovery Guide* is all practical. Through a series of questions, suggestions, brief essays, and exercises in imagination, you'll be guided to identify and clarify your goals for optimal vitality and health. It's designed to provide a boost to your efforts in creating the best life possible for yourself. While you can use it on your own, it's ideally used with a small group of supportive friends with similar interests. Enjoy!

CPSIA information can be obtained at www.ICGtesting.com
Printed in the USA
LVOW081911220512

282783LV00002B/18/P